ABOVE
AND
BEYOND

*Create a culture of engagement
and lead your dental team*

*High Impact Systems That Will
Transform Your Practice*

JANET STEWARD

ISBN: 1494367130
ISBN 13: 9781494367138

Library of Congress Control Number: 2013922286
CreateSpace Independent Publishing Platform
North Charleston, South Carolina

TABLE OF CONTENTS

ACKNOWLEDGEMENTS

There are so many people to give thanks and tribute to for helping to make this book happen. To Larry, my husband, thank you for always having faith in me and for your steadfast love and encouragement. Without you none of this would have been possible. For Geoff Engelhardt, DDS who has taught me so much about leadership, honor and integrity. For Chad Harris, DMD, my longest client and good friend who once told me that he was a businessman who happened to be a dentist and opened my eyes to the value within that statement. For my dear friend John Garlick, DDS a humble man of high principles, goodness, and decency – a true prince amongst men. And to all my clients past, present and future who have graciously invited me into their practices and their homes, become my friends, and shown me so much along the way.

Thank you.

DEDICATION

To my husband, Larry, I love you. This one's for you!

SECTION I

Why Don't They Just Do Their Jobs?

Ah, the sad lament of many a dentist. The reasoning is, if the team members would just do their jobs, and get along with one another, then the practice would be profitable and they could focus on the art of dentistry. However the problem is not that simple.

CHAPTER 1

THE DENTIST LEADERSHIP DILEMMA

What high-performing companies should be striving to create: A great place for great people to do great work.
— Marilyn Carlson, former CEO of Carlson Companies

Dentistry can be a lonely and somewhat isolated profession. If you are a dentist who owns your own practice, the frustrations are all too familiar. Does this sound like you? As your practice became established, and as your schedule began to fill with patients, you found yourself with much less time to focus on administrative concerns. Soon the number of business management issues requiring your attention began to multiply exponentially. In no time at all your business became "stuck," seemingly unable to grow beyond the rate afforded you by annual patient fee increases.

If you feel this way, you are not alone. My nationwide research study of more than 200 dentists (as reported in my 2007 book, *What Do Dentists Really Want?*), revealed a Catch-22 problem that I now call "The Dentist Leadership Dilemma": dentists own their own practices so they can have freedom and control over their own dentistry, but this same freedom often straddles them with business and management responsibilities that many dentists do not do well and most do not enjoy.

The way to solve this Catch-22 problem is to create an above and beyond team that gives the dentist control, cash flow, and time to enjoy it. The main message of my book is that any practice that cannot deliver all three is not worth owning. You can substantially increase your revenue and reduce your stress by becoming a more focused team leader. That is the first link on a four-link chain of profitability. This book provides a proven method that will allow you to do what you do best — practice the art of dentistry — and delegate the authority and responsibility for the rest.

Obviously the hardest part about owning a dental practice is that you can work so hard and get so little in return. That was the plight of a dentist in the Midwest, whose story illustrates my main message.

Stephen's Story

I will never forget the day when I met a decent, down-to-earth dentist named Stephen (real story, but not the real names). He had spent the last forty years as a dentist and he was still struggling. First there were the family issues. His daughter Amy was born three months premature with birth defects and to make matters worse, his wife suffered a stroke during the delivery. His wife survived, but required extra care. Amy, a sweet child, had thick glasses and difficulty in walking, but managed to get around with either a walker or a wheel-chair. What the family did have going for them was a second home by a lake, where the daughter could enjoy boating and horseback riding.

Stephen's second problem was his practice. To earn enough Stephen was having to work long hours, which kept him away from giving the time that his wife and daughter needed. He would not delegate anything, including charging and collecting money. He was so good hearted he often would not charge a patient, but would cut side deals to let them do some chore like fix his fence. His lack of delegation was driving his team nuts. Despite his lack of delegation, Stephen seemed to have a total inattention to practice details, which even allowed his office manager to embezzle substantial sums from him over the years.

Stephen did not have enough time for his wife and daughter and he also did not have enough cash to finish developing his practice. He had started building another treatment room that he needed to use to bring in a dental hygienist, but he could not afford to equip and finish the room. Stephen was in danger of losing the lake house, the one part of their life that brought joy to the family. He felt stuck in his mind and in his practice.

With our help Stephen was able to get unstuck. He turned his practice from a bunch of strugglers into an above and beyond team. His newfound leadership created a team commitment to improving the practice. This resulted in increased patient loyalty, which ulti-mately leads to increased profitability. Stephen was able to spend more time on what he loved doing, improving people's oral health, and less time with the nitty-gritty details of serving patients.

He also was able to save the lake house and spend more time with his disabled wife and daughter.

The secret was changing a struggling team into an above and beyond team, which can be better grasped when you know the five types of teamwork that exist at dental practices.

Worth Quoting

"If you work in an urgent-only culture, the only solution is to make the right things urgent."

Seth Godin, author of *Linchpin*

The Five Quintiles of Teamwork

Based on my over twenty-year track record of helping practices develop teamwork, I have developed a rating scale that is divided into five parts or quintiles. The teamwork at any practice can be rated on a spectrum from negative ten to positive ten. It would be a mistake to think that the lowest rating a practice could have is a one or a zero. There are many instances that the team commitment is in negative territory. That is hurting patient loyalty and lowering profitability. By my estimates, dental practices in America are about equally divided among the quintiles.

Lowest Quintile	Second Lowest Quintile	Middle Quintile	Second Highest Quintile	Highest Quintile
Teamwork Score -10 to -6	Teamwork Score -6 to -2	Teamwork Score -2 to 2	Teamwork Score 2 to 6	Teamwork Score 6 to 10
Turmoil Team	Troubled Team	Struggling Team	Adequate Team	Above and Beyond Team

The chart characterizes the five levels (quintiles) of teamwork where dentist offices typically function. How does your practice measure up?

Lowest Quintile (teamwork score of -10 to -6). This is a Turmoil Team. Typically there are open arguments between the dentist, hygienists, assistants, and office staff. There is constant patient turnover. Patients almost never refer family, friends, or coworkers.

Second Lowest Quintile (teamwork score of -6 to -2). This is a Troubled Team. Occasionally disagreements can flare up into open arguments between the dentist, hygienists, assistants, and office staff. Patients rarely make referrals.

Middle Quintile (teamwork score of -2 to 2). This is a Struggling Team. The patient experience can be hit or miss. Mostly the team members do their jobs. Occasionally patients make referrals.

Second Highest Quintile (teamwork score of 2 to 6). This is an Adequate Team. The office generally runs smoothly. Usually team members do their jobs. Patients have a generally good experience. More often than not patients will remain loyal and refer some others.

Highest Quintile (teamwork score of 6 to 10). This is an Above and Beyond Team. The practice runs like a well-oiled machine. Leadership is shared within the team, reducing the leadership load on the dentist. Every member knows their job and, where possible, has been cross-trained on the jobs of others. The office has a positive atmosphere that patients love. Patients are fiercely loyal. They feel blessed to have found the practice and are generous in referring others. Team members don't just do their jobs, they go above and beyond.

Here is the full quintile chart for the practice to use.

			Area		
Area	-10	-5	0	+5	+10
Greet patients by name	Never. Either don't care or too busy. Make them sign in	Seldom. Hit and miss.	Sometimes. We try but only with those we know	Mostly. Except if we're busy or don't know them	Always. Stop what we're doing and engage with a smile
	-10 -9 -8 -7	-6 -5 -4 -3	-2 -1 0 +1 +2	+3 +4 +5 +6	+7 +8 +9 +10
Keep patients waiting	Don't care about patients time	Patients jammed into the schedule willy nilly	It's about 50/50	We try but sometimes run behind	Well planned schedule, 95% seen on time
	-10 -9 -8 -7	-6 -5 -4 -3	-2 -1 0 +1 +2	+3 +4 +5 +6	+7 +8 +9 +10
Explain Treatment to patient	Patients lack clarity, knowledge and fee information	We do if we have time. Pretty hit and miss	Doctor never does, assistant/hygienist does sometimes.	Most of the time. Some people still leave not knowing.	Thoroughly educate all patients on treatment and costs
	-10 -9 -8 -7	-6 -5 -4 -3	-2 -1 0 +1 +2	+3 +4 +5 +6	+7 +8 +9 +10
Team atmosphere	No teamwork, no cooperation, lots of bickering and fighting	Occasional flareups, lack of communication.	Everyone pretty much out there for themselves	Look out for others, pitch in where possible	Cohesive, cooperative family feeling
	-10 -9 -8 -7	-6 -5 -4 -3	-2 -1 0 +1 +2	+3 +4 +5 +6	+7 +8 +9 +10
Policies and procedures in place	No written policies, chaotic	Everybody does their own thing, lack of cohesiveness	Some policies, most not revisited recently	Most policies in place. Mostly followed.	Everything is systemized and people follow the systems
	-10 -9 -8 -7	-6 -5 -4 -3	-2 -1 0 +1 +2	+3 +4 +5 +6	+7 +8 +9 +10
Patient loyalty	Patients never refer others	Patients seldom refer to us	Patients sometimes refer to us	Patients generally refer to us	Patients are our greatest fans and refer frequently
	-10 -9 -8 -7	-6 -5 -4 -3	-2 -1 0 +1 +2	+3 +4 +5 +6	+7 +8 +9 +10
Caring attitude with patients	Complete lack of interest in patients	Engage with patients we like	Somewhat engaged	Engage in small talk and some patient education	100% engaged, caring team
	-10 -9 -8 -7	-6 -5 -4 -3	-2 -1 0 +1 +2	+3 +4 +5 +6	+7 +8 +9 +10

My Quest to Create Above and Beyond Teams

I have worked in dentistry since 1989, and I began my dental practice management consulting career in 1999. In my early years I was very excited because consulting invariably led to immediate and dramatic successes in doctor, staff and patient satisfaction. Profitability was up and missed appointments were down. Staff and doctor morale was high and many of the staff issues that can drive a dentist crazy were really minimized or eliminated altogether.

Over the years I have always loved working with clients, so I made it a habit to check in with most of them over time, even long after the consulting process was completed, just to stay in touch. It has always been delightful to hear from the dentists whose practices have continued to thrive and grow. However, I became aware that this picture was not always rosy for every practice. Some, albeit a minority, were no better off a year or two after the consultation had ended than they had been before the process began. Doctor, staff and patient satisfaction had deteriorated, sometimes to the point the doctor would confide that he or she was thoroughly frustrated with the fact that he/she seemed unable to keep the momentum going.

I loved working with and following up with my engaged, successful clients, but I had to face the fact that this minority of clients was losing their proverbial mojo over time.

I knew there had to be a better way.

I began to study those engaged and successful clients of mine to see what it was that they had in common that was missing in those who were not enjoying the same kind of success. While I can speak for hours on the subject, I can distill it down to one core concept: the successful dentists lead, motivate, and care about their team members. This in turn creates a top quintile practice, the desired Above and Beyond Team.

Thus began my own journey of discovery. Countless books and seminars down the road and even a magical Leadership Excellence training course at the Disney Institute, and my journey still continues. I now enthusiastically teach what I've learned to my clients, especially the engaged and successful ones who are eager to take their practices to the next level. The transformations I have seen have been remarkable and, I am very happy to report, are beyond my greatest expectations.

What does an Above and Beyond Team look like? Instead of the team consisting of individual silos of good people, there is incredible cohesiveness where each person does their job in such a way that they set the next person up for success. Built into every day there's innovation, there's harmony, and there's the fun of meeting a challenge.

These practices don't have to focus on profitability in order to achieve it. Actually the potential for greater gains far exceeds what can be accomplished through profitability-focused leadership alone. People look forward to coming to work every day. Everyone is pulling towards a collective goal. They're having fun again. And, so am I.

You can too, as will be explained in the next chapter.

Worth Quoting

"There are only three measurements that tell you nearly everything you need to know about your organization's overall performance: employee engagement, customer satisfaction, and cash flow...It goes without saying that no company, small or large, can win over the long run without energized employees who believe in the mission and understand how to achieve it..."

Jack Welch, former CEO of GE

CHAPTER 2

THE BETTER SOLUTION: THE ABOVE AND BEYOND TEAM MODEL

The most dangerous leadership myth is that leaders are born-that there is a genetic factor to leadership. That's nonsense; in fact, the opposite is true. Leaders are made rather than born.

—Warren Bennis

If what dentists really want is profitability (remember, cash flow and time to enjoy it), why is the focus of this book on teamwork?

For years, when it comes to growing dental practices, the focus has been on increasing profitability. Systems are created, policies and procedures written and management systems are put in place. These initiatives frequently lead to an increase in profitability. The team is fired up in the initial stages of the process and the doctor is usually only too happy that someone has come along that can "fix" the practice. That way he or she can direct their focus to what they love most: delivering exceptional clinical care.

However, I've found this traditional approach has a downside that often results in a lack of sustainability. There is an erosion of long-term systems implementation and the ability to maintain growth for the practice. While the doctor is focused on delivering clinical care, the team's enthusiasm begins to wane since there is no leader and champion for the cause.

While normal staff turnover is a fact of life, when that happens systems become further diluted. Add to that the natural pull of the status quo which, just like the force of gravity, tends to, over time, also diminish systems. Gradually the doctor realizes that much of the effort, time, and resources may have been wasted because the system is no longer sustainable.

There are always exceptions to the rule and, almost invariably, those exceptions occur in practices where there is focused leadership that ensures sustainability. Of all the people that come and go in a practice, the one constant is the doctor, so why not focus on making the doctor an effective team leader? Once that's in place, you have the tools for developing an Above and Beyond Team. The shared leadership of an Above and Beyond Team guarantees a committed team that is collectively focused on the goals for the practice.

Certainly, there may be people that leave over time, but there are two factors that help maintain longevity and sustainability: a focused leader and an above and beyond culture. These two factors translate into a team that is on board, dialed in, and excited to be a part of an above and beyond practice. New team members that are added are immediately immersed in the goals and the culture of the practice and, with constant reinforcement from the leader, this synergy will be kept alive.

This does *not* mean that the doctors have to spend countless hours micromanaging the team. In fact, the more successful the leader and the greater the level of leadership throughout the team, the less time needs to be spent micromanaging day to day operations. Leadership should not rest solely at the top with the doctor but rather be developed throughout the team.

Is Team Leadership Innate?

Thankfully not, because that would mean that those lucky enough to have been born with the gene have it made, while the rest of us are destined to the life of being a follower with no hope of becoming leaders in our own right.

As people grow and mature, successful leaders tend to develop leadership qualities along the way. Perhaps they were troop leaders in the Girl Scouts or Boy Scouts, perhaps they were class president at school, or perhaps they were the captain of a sports team. They have often been placed in leadership roles in in the past. These all help to develop a foundation of good leadership qualities. What makes the difference, and turns mediocre leaders into successful ones, is a passion to keep honing these skills.

Great leaders set themselves apart from the rest of the pack by embarking on a never-ending journey of honing their skills through reading, studying, training, and continually adding to their own life experiences. They never lose sight of the goal of becoming a great leader and they pursue this passion throughout their lives. It's this specific, laser-like focus on improving their skills that propels them from good to great.

So What Is Team Leadership *Really?*

Leadership is a process whereby an individual influences a group of individuals to achieve a common goal.

The important first step lies in developing a solid grasp of who you are and where your strengths and weaknesses lie. Even the best leaders on the planet don't have strengths in every single area. It's important to know where your strengths lie and to make a disciplined effort to develop and expand upon those strengths. It's equally important to realize where your gaps lie and to have a systematic approach for filling in those gaps, sometimes turning them into strengths and sometimes working around them.

Remember, that it is your followers who determine whether or not you are successful. You have to convince your followers that you are *worthy* of being followed. We really have to focus on walking the walk because, as leaders, we tend to judge our leadership abilities by what we *intend* to do, whereas our followers judge us by our *actions*. There's no room in this equation for 'do as I say not as I do'. Successful leaders lead through their own actions first and foremost because it's these actions that inspire their followers. This is called leadership by example.

Followers choose to follow a leader for two reasons: respect and direction. If they don't respect your trustworthiness or integrity it will be tough to get them to follow you anywhere. They need a clear direction and they need to know what's expected of them and to be able to clearly visualize the goal. Everything you do communicates who you are; whether you are honorable and trustworthy or merely self-serving. Teams who have self-serving leaders do not follow them willingly; they simply obey them because they have to. They are the ones who seem checked out, they come to work but leave their hearts at the door. Your goal as a leader is for them to care enough to put their hearts into their work.

The first goal is to meet your people where they are and an important component of that is getting to know them as individuals. Unless you first get to know and care about them as individuals, it will be a challenge to get them to follow you to where you want them to go. To quote Teddy Roosevelt: *"People don't care how much you know until they know how much you care."* It goes beyond scratching the surface. It means getting to know about their families, their hobbies, what they're passionate about, and what challenges they have.

Worth Quoting

"Outstanding leaders go out of their way to boost the self-esteem of their personnel. If people believe in themselves, it's amazing what they can accomplish."

Sam Walton

I'm a people person so remembering what people tell me about their personal lives when I'm in a practice is something that comes pretty naturally to me. When I see them the next time, even if it is months later, I ask them about their kid, their dog, their new road bike, whatever it may be, it makes an impression. It tells them I am really interested and that I truly care about them as individuals. It can't be faked. If you don't care about them, don't expect them to care about you. This skill that can be developed and improved upon.

The next step is to develop a vision for the future for your practice and to be able to articulate your vision with conviction and passion and set the example for your team by living that vision every day. Your team will be watching you for clues to see if you are truly willing to walk the walk and talk the talk. If you do, they will too. If you do not, they won't. As Gandhi said: "We must become the change we want to see."

Worth Quoting

"Leadership is lifting a person's vision to high sights, the raising of a person's performance to a higher standard, the building of a personality beyond its normal limitations."

Peter Drucker

The Above and Beyond Team Leader in Action

Successful leaders are the driving force of change within an organization. An Above and Beyond Team Leader is a dentist who:

1. *Creates a Compelling Vision* for the future that inspires everyone on the team so that they put forth the maximum effort every day and love doing it.
2. *Organizes the Operation* by determining what needs to be done and making sure that everyone is going in the right direction with the right set of marching orders specific to their position.
3. *Motivates the Team* by involving everyone on the team so that they are committed to, and take ownership of, their part in the process.
4. *Commits to the Results* by creating accountability for himself/herself and the team to ensure the project moves forward towards the desired outcome.

Where We Are Headed in Section Two

FOCUSED	TEAM	PATIENT	INCREASED
LEADERSHIP	COMMITMENT	LOYALTY	PROFITABILITY

There are four links in the chain in the Above and Beyond Team Model. A chapter in section two will be devoted to examining these links in detail.

The First Link: Focused Leadership. The leader must focus on creating a team who is committed to the practice, the patients and one another. The leader must create a compelling vision, communicate that vision to the team, and keep the vision alive.

The Second Link: Committed Team. Why emotionally intelligent leadership is vital to creating team commitment, how emotional intelligence works in action, and what strategies work best.

The Third Link: Loyal Patients. Patients who keep their appointments, accept your treatment recommendations and act as advocates for your practice.

The Fourth Link: Increased Profitability. The payoff comes when all of the above finally culminate into increased profitability.

For the full discussion on how high performing teams can maximize profitability, please proceed to section two.

Above and Beyond Action Items

To create an Above and Beyond Team,
the dentist will:

- Identify his or her strengths and weaknesses.
- Get to know the staff – Remember that if you don't care about them, you can't expect them to care about you.
- Create a compelling vision to lead the team.

SECTION II

The Four Links to Success

To acquire something of value, there is a price that has to be paid. For a high performing team that maximizes practice profitability, the price is forging a chain that links together compelling vision, a committed team, loyal patients, and increased profitability.

CHAPTER 3

THE FIRST LINK: FOCUSED LEADERSHIP

If you want to build a ship, don't herd people together to collect wood and don't assign them tasks and work, but rather teach them to long for the endless immensity of the sea.

— Antoine de Saint-Exupery

There is a high correlation between successful leaders, strategic action, and results. It all starts with focused leadership. An often overlooked, yet extremely critical, aspect of leadership is the role of your vision for the future. It's essential to know the destination before you can navigate to it. Therefore, it is vital to decide where it is you want to take your practice before you can bring your Above and Beyond Team along for the journey.

The leader starts by creating a simple yet compelling vision and remains committed to making that vision a reality. The first two links in the chain ultimately lead to the final two links, which are loyal patients and greater profitability. How? The leader inspires the team with the vision and keeps it alive every day. The team will be given a clear blueprint for their own individual roles and responsibilities, will be provided with coaching and support, and will be motivated by feedback and praise. This will have a dramatic effect on the team and cause them to deliver an extraordinary experience for their patients. This experience will resonate with patients and motivate them to return and refer their friends.

There are, of course, many leaders who focus on greater profitability first without addressing the other links in the chain. While it is possible with this approach that they will achieve a temporary boost in profitability, there is a price to be paid. I find that the type of leader who insists on jumping to the last link is often one who leads through a demanding and commanding style. Or sometimes these leaders are passive, stating things once and wondering why the team doesn't follow through. While these leadership styles can generate bottom-line results, there are three things that they typically result in:

1. The leader is not a true leader because he has no willing followers; his team follows him because he demands that they do so.
2. His team is not engaged. They come in to work and they do what is expected but they leave their hearts at the door.
3. Because the team is not engaged, they do not have the energy or inclination to commit to an outstanding experience for their patients. They may even do a good job but being good can often be the greatest enemy of being excellent. If the team thinks they're doing a good enough job there is no motivation to get any better.

Instead, great leaders make it their mission to create a vision and to stay focused on that vision even while working through less than ideal situations. Instead of waiting for circumstances to be perfect, they establish the vision first and it becomes their guiding compass.

They set clear expectations for the team. They hire the right people, they inspire, and they create commitment from their team and loyalty from their patients, which ultimately results in greater profitability. Let's take a look at how you can become a great leader too, starting with creating *your* compelling vision.

Worth Quoting

"A leader has the vision and conviction that a dream can be achieved.
He inspires the power and energy to get it done."

Ralph Lauren

Step 1: Creating and Communicating a Compelling Vision

Leaders are responsible for developing and communicating a compelling vision of how they see their practices five or ten years in the future. It sets the tone and culture of the organization. It helps to attract and retain talented people. A powerful vision creates a shared purpose that resonates with people within the organization. It sets the direction for the team and communicates the values of the practice.

You may feel like you already have a vision statement. You may even have something on your website right now describing your practice's vision. Here's what most practices have: *...to be the leading dental practice and to deliver the best ... blah blah blah value... and deliver... blah blah blah customer service... blah blah blah.* After about the first five words of hearing that vision statement most people will have zoned out. I can just hear them saying, *Yeah, yeah, blah, blah, I've hear that about a million times....* Let's get real with your vision statement, let's make it dynamic, relevant and meaningful.

First, let's take a look at the difference between a vision and a mission statement.

Let's examine the purpose of a **mission statement**:

- It defines the present state or purpose of the practice.
- It answers three questions about why the practice exists: *What* the practice does, *Who* does it, and *How* it does what it does.
- It is longer than a vision statement and is written in a couple of sentences.
- Mission statements can change based on changing business realities.
- It gives teams a better perspective on how their position contributes to achieving the mission and can increase the level of productivity and engagement.

Examples:
ASPCA: The ASPCA Animal Behavior Center is dedicated to promoting balanced, respectful and enriched relations between people and pets through graduate and post-graduate programs for aspiring animal behaviorists; continuing behavioral education for shelter personnel, trainers, veterinarians, and other animal professionals; and the provision of practical, humane advice on pet behavior for owners.

Walt Disney Company: The mission of The Walt Disney Company is to be one of the world's leading producers and providers of entertainment and information. Using our portfolio of brands to differentiate our content, services and consumer products, we seek to develop the most creative, innovative and profitable entertainment experiences and related products in the world.

Citigroup: Our goal for Citigroup is to be the most respected global financial services company. Like any other public company, we're obligated to deliver profits and growth to our shareholders. Of equal importance is to deliver those profits and generate growth responsibly.

A mission statement serves a purpose but right now we need to focus on the vision statement. Instead of just a description, create something that touches your hearts, something that conjures up an emotion. Let's examine what a **vision statement** does:

- It defines what the practice wants to achieve.
- It provides inspiration and guidance on the focus of the practice in five or ten years and beyond.
- It becomes "true north" and helps the team to understand that, what they do every day, directly contributes to that goal.
- It is succinct (5-10 words), powerful, inspirational, and is easy for the team to learn and repeat at any given moment.

Examples:

Oxfam: A just world without poverty
Alzheimer's Association: Our vision is a world without Alzheimer's
Habitat for Humanity: A world where everyone has a decent place to live
Caterpillar: To be the global leader in customer service

Walt Disney Corporation: To make people happy
WalMart: To help people save money so they can live better

There are many excuses why practices do not have a written vision statement. For example:
- *We'll never get everyone to agree.*
- *It takes too long to develop.*
- *We know how to do our jobs already so what's the point?*
- *We'll get too much resistance.*
- *It'll get written and then sit on a shelf and become meaningless.*

While these may all be valid concerns, the benefits far outweigh the objections. If you can't envision where your practice is going, how will you align your team towards a successful future? If you don't know where you're going, how will you know when you've got there?

Worth Quoting

"If you limit your choices only to what seems possible or reasonable, you disconnect yourself from what you truly want, and all that is left is a compromise."

Robert Fritz

Strategies for Creating Your Vision

Envision the future. Start off by asking yourself some key questions such as:

- If you had no restrictions, what would you want your practice to look like in five or ten year's time?
- How would it be for you, for your team, and for your patients?
- What would it *feel* like?
- What would it *look* like?

Write two sentences that start off with the words "I believe..." or "I envision..." These words do not have to stay there and can be taken out later. Don't put the obvious what you do (practice dentistry) in the vision.

Creating the vision statement. You don't have to do this all at once but be sure you set aside the time to devote to this critical step.

It's important *not* to start off with trying to write the vision statement perfectly right from the get go. A better way is to start off by doing a little brainstorming and thinking about how you want your patients to feel (in 5-10 years) and how you want your Above and Beyond Team to look. Try writing down some key words, words that are powerful and have emotion attached.

Be sure to work on this by yourself. Too much input from others can be very confusing and really muddy the waters of your thought process. As the leader, you play the greatest part in developing your vision. This is *your* practice—therefore, the vision has to resonate with *you* first and foremost. Take the time to create your vision statement free from the input of other members of the team. It is possible, once the vision has been crafted, that you may get additional ideas from your team that you would like to incorporate but, for the most part, your vision should be complete when you present it to them.

The vision statement should be short, simple, and concise. It should be no more than 8-10 words (15 at the most), the shorter the better. It should be patient-centered, team centered and carry a compelling, emotional message.

For example, I was talking with a dentist in Colorado about how he envisioned the future of his practice. We brainstormed words that described how he wanted the practice to look and feel. His first desire was that the patients feel that they had received the *ultimate* experience. But his biggest concern was that everyone in the office was working as a seamless team, which was not the current reality. Thinking over these concepts, we found the right sentence to encapsulate his vision.

We are a team, committed to creating remarkable patient experiences.

Here are some other real examples from dental practices I've worked with:

- *"Where patients leave feeling like family."*
- *"Providing our patients with the best experience from beginning to end."*
- *"Changing the way you think about going to the dentist by being present and engaged at all levels."*
- *"Striving for perfection and settling for excellence."*
- *"The patient experience redefined."*
- *"Creating moments of magic for our patients."*
- *"Putting our patients at the center of everything we do."*
- *"Creating extraordinary patient experiences by recognizing and rewarding individual team initiative."*

Worth Quoting

"The greatest danger for most of us is not that our
aim is too high and we miss it,
but that it is too low and we reach it."

Michelangelo

Communicating the Vision:
Communicating your vision is an important event, so pick the time
and place for this moment carefully. It should be in a meeting that
is separate from a routine staff meeting, preferably a meeting just to
address the vision, after all it is not an afterthought but a pivotal, defining
moment for your practice. What you have to say will guide the
future of the practice and shouldn't be buried within a regular meeting
so that the importance is lost. Allow enough time for the team to
absorb and discuss the vision for the future of the organization, how it
resonates with each of them and what it means to the practice and the
patients. Encourage feedback and discussion after your presentation.

Here are the four steps you need for communicating the vision to
your team.

1. **Vision:** Lead off by laying out your vision in a clear and concise manner.
    Start off by framing the vision statement first, using language
    that comes from the heart. Why is the vision so important to you?
    What about the vision excites you the most. How will the vision feel
    to your team and to your patients once the goal is reached?

2. **Reality:** This statement outlines why this awesome vision is not yet a reality. What are the barriers and obstacles that are preventing the vision from becoming a reality?

3. **Reshaping:** What changes need to take place in order for the goals outlined in the vision to be reached? What are the changes that are needed to transform the practice from your current reality to the new reality outlined in the vision?

4. **Call to Action:** Here's how you're going to make the change a reality. Give the team one specific call to action that they can begin implementing right away. Remember how Mayor Giuliani used eradicating graffiti as one of his steps towards reinventing New York? How simple, yet stunningly effective, was that?

As an example, I'll return to the dentist I just described above. Here is how he communicated his compelling vision in an effort to create an Above and Beyond Team.

1. **Vision:** *We are a team, committed to creating remarkable patient experiences.*
    This practice was a merger of two practices that had never really solidified into one cohesive team. They still operated as individuals instead of operating as a cohesive unit and it created conflict. When communicating this vision to the members of the team, the dentists spoke from the heart about why this was so important to them.

    One dentist said to the group, "We haven't always been a team and we know this has been difficult for everyone. We haven't lived this vision, but this is where we want to be, this is where we're going. We're 100% committed to this vision."

2. **Reality:** Again, the dentists acknowledged the current situation they were seeing, that they were a group of individuals, each with great strengths, but lacking the ability to work together. "We are good people," they said, "but we are not a team. It's almost like we are a bunch of silos, albeit good silos. Now we need to take the next step and get out of our silos and become one practice."

3. **Reshaping:** The dentists expressed what changes they felt were necessary to make the vision the new reality. They told the group, "We need to look for creative ways for us all to become part of this team behind the vision."

4. **Call to Action:** The last step was to express how they would be leading the charge by living these changes themselves and asking each of them to take action as well. The key of the message was that "each one of us is charged with setting each other up for success." In other words, you can't think of yourself as an island and only do what is best for you. Everything you do should also be helping those around you succeed.

The final step in communicating the vision is to allow time for a discussion with the group. Give them time to digest and warm up to your vision and call to action. Ask them what their reactions are to this vision. How does it make them feel? Sometimes you will be met with silence because no one wants to be the first to speak. If this is the case, tell them you want to go around the room and hear from each person about what they think. This is a good opportunity to reiterate the call to action.

With most teams, you will get a variety of these responses.

- Defensive: "Well I feel like we are doing a pretty good job of being a team."
- Supportive: "We've had so much conflict in this practice in the last few years. This is a great vision."
- Guarded: "I'm not sure – I haven't had time to process it."
- Skeptical: "This is never going to work for our team."

Regardless of the responses you receive, remember that in no way should they alter your course of action. In a later section we'll discuss how to address the situation when someone on the team refuses to come into alignment with the new vision. For now, work on making the vision come alive.

Making the Vision Come Alive

Communicating your vision and ensuring that it is remains the focus into the future, is a *process*, not an event. This is not something that is done in one single meeting or only at staff meetings. Instead, it's communicated every day through words and deeds with you, the leader, being the greatest champion of all. Now that you have created the vision and inspired and motivated your team with that vision, it is time to start making it a part of the DNA of the practice.

Lead with Passion: Excitement from the leader is infectious. Let your team see, feel, and hear your passion for the destination you have mapped out. Demonstrate the behavior that you would like to see from them. Live the vision through your actions so that it becomes more than just words but rather a way of life, an expectation of everyone on the team with nothing less being accepted.

Meetings: Whenever you get together for any kind of meeting, such as one-on-one meetings with a team member, performance appraisals, morning meetings, team huddles, or staff meetings, find ways to reiterate your vision. Talk more at length about what that vision means to your practice, your team, and your patients. Identify actions and behavior that support the vision. You and your team should be able to recite it if you are woken up at 2:00 am. Include an agenda item for each staff meeting that asks for ways in which individual team members have lived the vision in the past day/week/month.

Recognition and Reward: Go for a positive approach. Instead of looking for ways in which the vision is *not* being supported, look for ways that it *is*. Have team members identify specific behaviors being done by others that are aligned with the vision. Have team members recognize one another in meetings and reward both of them for their efforts to promote teamwork and live the vision.

Success Stories: Share success stories and progress you have made towards reaching your goals. Regular updates and team recognition should never be underestimated. *The most* meaningful thing to an employee is to feel recognized and valued. This has been proven through numerous studies both nationally and worldwide.

Patient Feedback: Focus on taking patient feedback seriously and sharing it with the team. There are several different types of software systems available that include patient surveys into their menu of services such as Demand Force and Light House. In the Appendix there is an example of one that has worked very well for my clients. I especially like the open-ended questions for the important information that can sometimes be gleaned from patient responses.

Sharing both positive and negative feedback provides you with the opportunity to celebrate and brainstorm how to improve results through changing behaviors.

Display the Vision: The more your vision is shared, with patients and team members, the greater the probability of it becoming a reality. Put the vision on business cards, embed it in emails, and include it on stationery and appointment reminder cards. Create posters throughout the practice stating your vision.

Huddles: Finally, if there is just one call to action for perpetuating the vision, it would take place in the huddle. We will discuss this more in a later chapter, but briefly, the huddle leader states the vision or asks someone else to do it, *every* time. The huddle leader then asks for input from the team on what people have done recently to reach the vision. Additionally, reward any great ideas and write them into your policy so they can be implemented by the whole team.

Worth Quoting

"Goals. There's no telling what you can do when you get inspired by them.
There's no telling what you can do when you believe in them.
And there's no telling what will happen when you act upon them."

Jim Rohn

As the leader, you must be willing to put yourself out there. It's up to you as the dentist to be the first one to act. Do the things to keep the vision alive. Find something specific and tangible to help set someone up for success. Show the team that the vision is important to you and they will follow because they will be inspired and motivated.

Above and Beyond Action Items

Creating and communicating a compelling vision is a key first step in the journey. The dentist must:

- Envision the future he or she wants for the practice in five to ten years.
- Brainstorm emotionally impactful key words that resonate with this vision of the future
- Take time to draft a clear, concise vision statement that is patient-centered and team centered and carries a compelling, emotional message.
- Communicate your vision to the team – this is a crucial moment so choose the time and place carefully.
- Make the vision come alive by leading with passion; reiterating the vision at all meetings; using positive reinforcement; sharing success stories; focusing on patient feedback; displaying the vision in the office; and making it a key part of your daily huddle.

CHAPTER 4

THE SECOND LINK: COMMITTED TEAM

We are dangerous when we are not conscious of our responsibility for how we behave, think, and feel.
— Marshall B. Rosenberg

When I work with practices, I often find there is a clear disconnect between the dentist at the top and the staff working under him or her. There can be many factors involved in this, from the differences in education and motivation to a feeling that a certain amount of distance is the professional way to behave. Some dentists don't understand why there is any need to relate to their staff on a personal level at all.

But what I try to help my clients understand is that this emotional connection between the staff and the dentist is vital to having a top-notch practice. Showing a genuine interest in coworkers is the first step toward creating a practice that runs smoothly and empowers staff to work diligently to help everyone succeed.

Above and Beyond Teams care about each other and want to help one another.

Perhaps this seems silly to you? Let's take a look at why emotional intelligence is such a crucial part of the puzzle.

Why Emotional Intelligence Is So Vital to Individuals and Businesses

While IQ is a good predictor of your ability to get into college and get your degree, EQ (emotional intelligence) is a good predictor of your success in business, relationships, and life in general. It is estimated that 75 percent of careers that derail do so due to a lack of emotional intelligence. The Carnegie Institute of Technology indicates that 85 percent of financial success is due to what they term "human engineering," i.e., your ability to communicate, negotiate, and lead. Amazingly, only 15% is due to intelligence and technical knowledge.

So what is emotional intelligence anyway? Simply stated, it is the ability to tune into your own emotions and to get along with others. It is the ability to recognize your own emotions, control impulsive behaviors and feelings, tune into the emotions, concerns, and needs of others, to communicate with clarity and inspiration, and manage conflict and change.

Just like IQ, EQ (Emotional Intelligence) can also be measured. Certainly, the measure is not as tangible as those from a profit and loss statement, however, as my friend and mentor Mark LeBlanc says, "It's the intangibles that drive the tangibles."

> ## Worth Quoting
>
> "If your emotional abilities aren't in hand, if you don't have self-awareness, if you are not able to manage your distressing emotions, if you can't have empathy and have effective relationships, then no matter how smart you are, you are not going to get very far."
>
> Daniel Goleman

Why EQ in a Leader Is So Important

The significance of what a leader says and does cannot be under-estimated. People naturally watch and take their cues from their boss. An enthusiastic, empathetic, visionary leader has an incredible impact on the team's performance, as well as the bottom-line of the business. A leader who is not in tune with the needs and moods of the group, and by extension, the individuals within the group, leaves the group feeling fearful and anxious and can drag the entire organization into a downward spiral.

An emotionally intelligent leader knows that EQ leadership is not up to just one individual on the team but should rather be inspired and encouraged throughout the organization. In an organization, the leader is the one who begins the task of self-discovery and developing emotional intelligence. Then, with clarity and direction, the leader begins developing additional leaders throughout the organization. This is how you can move from micro-managing every aspect of your

41

practice to empowering your Above and Beyond Team to be able to effectively manage their own areas. The greater the emotional intelligence level of the leader and the group as a whole, the better people work together, and the better the environment within the organization becomes.

Great leaders recognize that an optimistic leader is confident and reassuring. Optimistic and reassuring leadership is a key factor in the success of an organization. As Napoleon succinctly stated: "A leader is a dealer in hope." One study estimates that for every one percent improvement in the climate of an organization, there is a 2 percent increase in revenue. Another study of cardiac care units where the nurses' general moods were unhappy and disgruntled shows that the death rate amongst patients was four times higher than in comparable units. While climate alone does not determine the performance of an organization, studies show that organizations where the group enjoys coming to work have 20 percent to 30 percent higher performance than other organizations. Creating a positive atmosphere of hope and optimism has a directly positive effect on the ultimate outcome.

Learning Centers of the Brain and Why You *Can* Change

It's important to understand the portion of the brain that controls one's emotions. The neocortex, or reasoning part of the brain, is responsible for "higher functions" such as sensory perception, generation of motor commands, spatial reasoning, conscious thought, and language. It is the newest part of the brain. When learning things such as new tasks or a new subject, this is the part of the brain that is responsible for learning and retaining that information. What the neocortex learns has a tendency to be forgotten unless the information is used and repeated. For example, one may learn a new language but, if it is not practiced repeatedly, many of the details are forgotten.

The limbic, or emotional part of the brain, on the other hand, supports a variety of functions, including emotion, behavior, motivation, and long-term memory. It appears to be primarily responsible for our emotional life, and has a great deal to do with the formation of memories. What is learned in the limbic region of the brain is best learned through research, practice, and feedback. As long as repetition is the key, what is learned in the limbic part of the brain can be retained for many years and indeed forever. In other words, the limbic part of the brain is where emotional intelligence resides.

This is good news for people who genuinely want to modify their behavior and learn a new way of doing things. With commitment and true desire, it can be accomplished. It requires a fair amount of bravery to assess one's own emotional intelligence and to come face to face with the realities of one's frailties. Likewise, it also takes courage to examine and question the culture within an organization and to determine what the guiding principles within the organization are. Not all of these principles are positive and constructive. Leaders are either in tune with the organization and the people in it or they are tuned out. Do you think you are a leader that "gets it" within your team?

Leaders that "get it"

1. These leaders, by definition, have a high degree of emotional intelligence.
2. They are able to understand their own behavior and manage their impulses and emotions.

3. They understand and have empathy for the individuals within the group.
4. They lead their teams with energy and enthusiasm.
5. They share their feelings and concerns and thereby model the behavior they would like to see from the group.
6. As a result, the team becomes motivated and finds their work both rewarding and meaningful.

Leaders that don't "get it"

1. They don't bond with their team.
2. The team shows up for work, but leave their hearts at the door.
3. Their leadership often results in fear, anger, apathy, and sullenness from their teams.
4. They are negative.
5. Sometimes, they can initially come across as charming and caring, however, it soon becomes apparent that this is just a pretense to get what they want since they filter everything through the lens of 'what's in it for me.'
6. Occasionally, these types of leaders can be happily ignorant of how their teams feel, unaware of the undercurrents that may exist.

Emotional Intelligence Strengths

Emotional Intelligence is not innate, but rather, is a learned behavior. Frequently, emotionally intelligent leaders have been exposed to leadership early in their lives. For example, they may have been a team captain, taught Sunday school, or coached Little League. Over time, these skills are often enhanced through life experiences, which help to broaden this foundation. No leader, however great he or she may be, has strengths in every area. Most great leaders have strengths in several of the following areas. With motivation and a desire to enhance their skills through identification, work and repetition, they are able to enhance their strengths as well as fill in some of the gaps.

The Four Aspects of Emotional Intelligence:

1. **Self Awareness:** People with a highly developed sense of self awareness understand their own emotions and moods and the impact that these tend to have on others. They have a firm grasp on their own strengths and weaknesses and, ultimately, tend to have greater self-confidence.
   a. *Recognition*: Competency in reading one's own emotions and recognizing the impact they have on others.
   b. *Strengths/Shortcomings*: Determine one's own strengths and recognize shortcomings.
   c. *Confidence*: Belief in one's own self worth and abilities.

2. **Self-Management:** The ability to control one's emotions, take initiative, adapt to changing situations, and follow through with commitments. People with high self-management skills are inclined to make better decisions. Instead of letting their emotions dictate their decisions, they think things through, weighing the pros and cons. They have a personal conversation going on in their heads: How will what I say be received? Does this fit my moral code of ethics? Am I being completely

honest? They are no longer a prisoner of their own emotions. They are less likely to be diverted and go off on tangents. It allows them to be calm, clear, and positive. Emotions are contagious and these positive emotions trickle down through the rest of the team.

   a. *Control:* Ability to control one's own disruptive emotions and impulses.

   b. *Values:* Display honesty, integrity, and trustworthiness.

   c. *Optimism:* Having a positive attitude.

3. **Social Awareness:** In a word, empathy. The ability to read the cues of body language, tone and pace, to help understand what drives others, and to get on their same wavelength. They are comfortable socially and tune into the dynamics of a group or organization. They are able to adapt so that what they say and do is appropriate to the individual and the situation. They can calm people that are anxious and joke and have fun with the team when appropriate. They are interested in hearing what people have to say. They're approachable. They consider other people's feelings. They tend to retain staff and generate loyalty and commitment.

   a. *Empathy:* Ability to understand and share the feelings of others.

   b. *Organizational empathy:* Ability to recognize and understand the culture and moods within the organization.

   c. *Needs:* Meet the needs of others.

4. **Relationship Management:** The ability to maintain good relationships and work well as part of a team. These people are able to persuade others in a compelling manner. They are able to manage conflicts and collaborate effectively. They are tuned into

their own emotions, the emotions of the team, and the mindset of the group. It goes beyond simply being friendly and evolves towards moving the team in the right direction with a powerful vision. People are drawn to them.

a. *Vision:* Create a compelling vision and get the team motivated to support that vision.
b. *Change:* Lead change within others and the organization.
c. *Conflict:* Skillfully resolve disagreements.
d. *Teamwork:* Develop teamwork through cooperation and collaboration.

Worth Quoting

"But once you are in that field, emotional intelligence emerges as a much stronger predictor of who will be most successful, because it is how we handle ourselves in our relationships that determines how well we do once we are in a given job."

Daniel Goleman

Implementation Strategies for Individuals

Now that we've reviewed the strengths that you want to cultivate, it is time to think about how to implement them. While it's exciting and inspiring to read the theory of emotional intelligence, the true magic begins when you start using it in your own life. It has often been said that people don't change but, when practice is combined with passion, amazing things happen. It's magical and exciting to see the changes occur and it will give you confidence to continue.

Implementation is where the proverbial rubber meets the road. Everything looks good in theory but, unless it can work in practice, that's all it ever is: a theory. The first essential step towards implementation is desire. It starts with an individual or team truly buying into the process, the benefits, and the desired outcome. These principles will need to be practiced repeatedly so that the limbic part of the brain literally becomes rewired.

Let's examine some practical steps to begin the journey in your own life.

1. **Self Evaluation**

   Take a good look at who you are. Right now. Today. Have you allowed your dreams to fade? Have your dwindling dreams allowed you to settle for something that no longer puts the wind in your sails? This is where you take stock of your strengths as well as your weaknesses. This is where you identify the gaps. This is where you compare who you have become with the vision you created in the last chapter.

   When it comes to self evaluation, it can be extremely helpful to gather insight from some trusted friends and coworkers. You need to speak with the people who are willing to give you honest feedback, both positive and negative.

It's not uncommon to find strengths that, when overused, become weaknesses. Be prepared to recognize and identify when this happens.

Focus on what you do well, as well as your shortcomings. Keep it balanced. If you don't, the exercise will be dishearteningly demotivating. Take a look at the emotional intelligence list of strengths and rate yourself. Ask yourself the following questions and be sure to write down your answers.

What are your greatest strengths?
What could use some improvement?
What are your emotional intelligence skills?
What skills could use some work and refinement?
What is not part of your skill set yet?

2. **Creating Sustainable Change**
   Decide what is the one most important emotional intelligence strength that *you* want to improve? It is really important to follow your *own* passion. This is really critical. No one else should tell you what you should work on. If it is important to you, it will get done. If it's important to someone else, it probably won't get done. It could be a strength that needs some improvement or it could be a strength that is lacking. It has to be a strength that you are excited about improving and/or changing. Your path towards change is one that will require effort on a daily basis so you had better be heading towards something that you are highly motivated to improve upon.

For example, let's take someone who wants to work on the skill of empathy. Let's say their mission is getting to know their team members better. They begin to find out what challenges the individuals face, both at work and personally. The leader learns what they love, what motivates them, what makes them tick. This knowledge helps him to identify with the team members, to see them through a different lens, to empathize with what's going on in their lives. It helps him to see the bigger picture and to relate on a far deeper level than he may have been able to do before. Furthermore, the leader begins to work on empathy outside of work as well. Instead of judging the beggar at the side of the road he chooses to see him through a different lens. The more you practice your skill in multiple areas of your life, the quicker the limbic brain becomes rewired until it no longer becomes an effort.

Here are some strategies to help you.
a. *Core Competency:* Determine the core competency you want to implement.
b. *Practice:* Find as many ways to practice as you can. That may involve communicating more effectively with a patient, being more nurturing in your personal relationships, or improving your coaching skills in Little League.
c. *Visualization:* Visualize yourself excelling at this core competency. Athletes often visualize catching the game winning touchdown, winning the race or performing a perfect dive. It provides another effective way of rewiring the limbic brain.
d. *Feedback:* Get feedback from the people you trust to give you both positive and negative feedback. Form teams who meet regularly to support one another.

Be patient. Old habits do not just magically disappear. Change requires commitment, practice and constant reminders. As the new behavior becomes a more robust pathway in the brain, the need for this level of focus diminishes over time until it requires no effort at all.

I worked with a dentist who tended to lash out in anger when upset. Here are the strategies we employed to redirect that weakness.
a. Don't jump in.
b. Step back and allow the other person to speak. Listen.
c. Be objective. Ask yourself if you're jumping to conclusions.
d. Ask clarifying questions.
e. Prepare proactively in advance if you suspect a trigger situation may arise. Plan how you will handle it.

The act of creating strategies that work for your own issue will help you to apply them consistently. Create a list of the steps you plan to take to improve. Write them down and keep them in a place you will see them every day. Let the magic begin!

Developing Emotional Intelligence at an Organizational Level

On an individual level, once you have assessed your own level of EQ strengths and weaknesses, the next step is to dive right into making change happen. There is an additional step when working with a group *before* the individuals within the group begin working on their own EQ.

The realities of the group culture need to be examined. This needs to take place before developing the compelling vision that will guide the team. On an individual level, the vision provides the energy and passion for change. In a group setting, the vision is no longer personal enough. The passion and energy created by a personal vision are not powerful enough to motivate change in a group. Once groups fully understand the realities of how they function, they are able to move to the next step of affecting change.

Groups, like one-on-one relationships, frequently have some level of dysfunction in the way they interact. Often the ground rules for communication have long been established, and even unconsciously, new team members adapt to and adopt these behaviors. It is imperative to uncover these types of unhealthy norms in order to begin the process of addressing them effectively.

Emotional intelligence qualities are the same for groups as they are for individuals: self awareness, self management, social awareness, and relationship management. The goal is to practice self awareness by taking note of the mood and needs of the group and responding with empathy. This very act will help to create positive norms such as listening, open and honest communication, and staying on track.

Groups tend to be smarter than individuals but only when their EQ competency level is high. The leader is the one who has the greatest influence in paving the way for the team. I have never encountered employees that decide to begin this process on their own without the leader first becoming the standard bearer.

Let's take a look at some of the benefits:

1. Teams who observe their leaders searching for the truth, feel safe in doing so themselves.
2. People are encouraged to be open and honest about topics they may previously have felt uncomfortable discussing.
3. Recognition alone of unhealthy norms is the first step in the process of creating change.

Group Evaluation

Group evaluation is an important initial step in the process of evaluating your strengths and weaknesses and the culture that actually exists within your practice. I believe this an area where a trained and experienced outside professional will be most beneficial. You can manage this process yourself, of course, but a professional can help you avoid the emotional and potentially destructive land mines inherent in this process.

If you decide to go it alone, it's very important to complete the self-assessment outlined above, and to be honestly committed to following through. If you are easily hurt by criticism or don't really care to hear what others think of you, then it's definitely appropriate to engage an experienced professional.

The purpose of the process is to hear the positives and negatives about your leadership and the culture within your practice.

The first step is to schedule a meeting a week or so in advance and let team members know that your goal is an open and honest discussion of the culture and leadership within the practice. Let them know that you're providing advance notice because everyone will be expected to contribute to the discussion. It's important to be prepared for the worst, even the potential emotional "train wreck" that can result when a group is given the opportunity to express pent up frustrations and work related issues that may have been ignored for years.

For the meeting, you'll need a large note pad or white board and magic markers. If you're going it alone, it's often best if you serve as the team scribe to record comments and feedback. It's important to listen appropriately and record comments accurately without getting defensive or argumentative. In fact, it's best not to respond at all, which can be quite a challenge when you feel strongly that the feedback is unfair or when you hear what you feel are blatant falsehoods. If you've decided on outside help, let that person facilitate the discussion and record the comments.

At the meeting, the process begins by asking the team for their ideas on what is positive about the practice and the group culture. You may get answers like: "We all like one another, we all participate and share our ideas," and "there's a lot of energy in our meetings." Write the answers down.

Next, ask what team members to list some of the more dysfunctional attributes within the practice and of the group. Here you may expect answers like: "We don't want to bring up mistakes for fear of hurting someone else in the group, we are afraid of voicing our opinion, great ideas discussed during our meetings are not followed up on," and, "our viewpoints do not seem to count." Write these answers down as well. This feedback is very important on your journey to improve your practice. It's helpful to remember that we judge ourselves by our intentions and others judge us by our behaviors. Whether we like it or not, all leaders are judged. Negative feedback helps us learn how others perceive our behaviors and give us the clues we need to make improvements.

Create Sustainable Change

Acknowledge your successes. You deserve it. Build upon and strive to improve these areas. Never underestimate the value of these accomplishments because, as you work on the second half of the list, your dysfunctions, you will need to draw upon these positive attributes.

Prioritize the list of dysfunctions and discuss tangible ways in which to turn them around. This becomes the road map for the group that will keep everyone heading in the same direction with the right set of marching orders. Begin working on the list strategically, one at a time. Follow your blueprint of strategies and, most importantly, keep them alive every day. Review them during your staff meetings. At the end of the staff meeting, evaluate how it went. Remember to celebrate the successes!

Conclusion

Remember that the great news is that EQ can be developed. Reading this is just one small step in the journey. Your commitment and dedication to the implementation process is the next step. Just like the idea of "If you build it, they will come," do this and you will reap rewards beyond anything you could have imagined.

Above and Beyond Action Items

Emotional Intelligence is vital to a successful doctor and practice. Here are the steps you can take to improve your EQ:

- Take the time to understand the importance of EQ in your leadership, the parts of the brain responsible for emotional intelligence, and why it is something you can truly improve upon and change.
- Review the emotional intelligence strengths: Self Awareness, Self Management, Social Awareness, and Relationship Management.
- Perform a self-evaluation by taking stock of your strengths and analyzing the gaps. Ask trusted friends and colleagues for honest feedback.
- Ask yourself the following questions and be sure to write down your answers:
    1. What are your greatest strengths?
    2. What could use some improvement?
    3. What are your emotional intelligence skills?
    4. What skills could use some work and refinement?
    5. What is not part of your skill set yet?

- Create sustainable change one area at a time. Start by choosing one thing to work on that you really want to improve.
- Evaluate the group culture of your practice in relation to the EQ strengths and then repeat the exercise as a group.
- Develop a plan for sustainable change in the group with clear action items.

CHAPTER 5

THE THIRD LINK: PATIENT LOYALTY

Loyal customers, they don't just come back, they don't simply recommend you, they insist that their friends do business with you.
— Chip Bell, Founder of Chip Bell Group

You might expect a chapter on patient loyalty to begin with a laundry list of all the ways you could create an amazing patient experience. I personally and wholeheartedly advocate for many strategies that have helped other practices achieve a better patient experience. Nonetheless, lists, no matter how exhaustive, don't lead to patient loyalty in and of themselves. Patient loyalty, and this is the crux of this chapter, springs from the team that is enthusiastic, engaged and passionate about what they do.

Since your team's actions determine the patient experience, many dentists with highly successful practices have concluded that the team should be treated as well, if not better, than your patients. Your first responsibility as a leader is to focus on the team experience, knowing that the team experience will eventually take your practice to the next level. Team loyalty translates to patient loyalty. If your team is committed to you and to your practice, you'll find the members of your team will do *anything* you ask *and more*. At this point, your team will be as motivated as you are to create the amazing Above and Beyond experience for your patients.

Later in this chapter you'll look at what most "bosses" think motivates their staff members, and compare that with staff members say is most important to them. For staff members, feeling appreciated ranks at the top of the list, while most bosses think money is the greatest motivator.

Why is it so important to create an Above and Beyond practice? There are several reasons. Profitability is, of course, one of them. The cost of marketing to generate new patients is extremely high. If your practice becomes an Above and Beyond practice, your existing patients will be your biggest advocates and actively encourage their friends, family and co-workers to seek you out for their dental needs. Not only is this free marketing, but patients that are referred by people they know, arrive in your practice with an already established level of trust, thereby setting the stage for a successful and long-term relationship with you.

Another reason why this is so important is that your patients are much more likely to follow your treatment recommendations. They will willingly schedule and keep their appointments for their hygiene visits and their trust in you makes them much more receptive to your restorative recommendations. They tend to have a far lower cancellation and no show level than similar patients in an average practice. Because they like you and are committed to your practice, they wouldn't dream of not showing up for their appointment and, if a scheduling conflict occurs, they are far more likely to call and give you adequate notice that they need to reschedule. And, finally, these patients pay their bills.

Lastly, because the retention rate of patients in your practice is so high and because they refer many of their friends, family, and coworkers into your practice, you will ultimately be able to weed out those people who are not your ideal patients. These patients who don't keep their appointments, don't refer their friends, and don't follow your treatment recommendations can be encouraged to seek their dental happiness elsewhere!

To be clear, not every practice has a business model that requires an Above and Beyond patient experience. There are plenty of very profitable, high volume, low to average patient retention practices that rely on advertising, insurance, and even sometimes Medicaid to fill their chairs. There is absolutely nothing wrong with this approach but, I'm guessing that, if you are reading this book, your practice is probably not one of those or you're considering changing that model and wondering how to do it. If the latter is the case, send me an email or give me a call and we can have a strategic conversation because the process needs to be approached in a calculated and well-planned manner.

This begs the question of why everyone doesn't create an Above and Beyond model. Because it's not that easy! It requires desire, planning, commitment, and discipline. It requires focused leadership. It requires a team that is totally, one hundred percent on board with you because, without that, it simply won't happen. It's a journey, not an event.

What does your team want?

Interestingly, what *you* think your team wants is not necessarily what *they* actually do want. Take a look at the table below. It lists, in order, what is important to your team and the order in which bosses think those things are important.

What Teams Need	Order of Team Priority	Order of Bosses' Priority
Feeling appreciated	1	8
Feeling "in" on things	2	10
Sympathetic help on personal problems	3	9
Job security	4	2
Good wages	5	1
Interesting work	6	5
Promotion/growth opportunities	7	3
Personal loyalty to workers	8	6
Good working conditions	9	4
Tactful discipline	10	7

Now *that's* eye-opening isn't it? Most bosses think that the number one most important thing to their teams is money but that actually ranks at a mere five out of ten. Of course that assumes that your workers are being paid a fair wage that is competitive with other practices in the area. Once that BAM (Bare Assed Minimum) has been met, money drops to a meager five out of ten. So, if you're thinking has always been that all your team wants is more money to keep them happy, now's the time to change that thinking. Let's take a closer look at each of the ten on the list of the needs of teams and look at them in greater depth.

1. *Feeling Appreciated*: When I began my career in dentistry managing a very profitable group practice, I had a boss who was really a decent guy. We all liked him and worked hard for him. While he did a fair job of trying to show us that he appreciated us, it was far from great. At the end of the day, as he was walking out of the door he would say, "Thanks guys, you all did a great job today." Not so bad, you may think. However, as I would later learn and studies would show, the impact of heartfelt, specifically targeted praise is exponentially more effective. Say, for example, had he said, "Janet, thank you for the way you handled Mrs. Jones today. She was so nervous but you tuned into that and talked her down and when she left she even commented that this was the best visit she had ever had. Nice job!" Specific praise, given in that manner, will make the recipient strive to do an even better job next time because they know exactly what is important. A great book on this subject is *Whale Done* written by Ken Blanchard. Pick up a copy, it will only take a couple of hours to read and will be well worth your time. I often get asked how busy dentists can possibly remember who to praise, when to give praise, and about what specifically. The way one of my clients solved that problem was to carry a small notebook and pen in his pocket so he could quickly jot down one or two words to remind himself. Clearly, since this is number one for teams, this is way too important to overlook.

2. *Feeling "In" On Things*: Meaning that they feel like their opinions matter, that they are included in what's going on in the practice, and that everyone is treated fairly. When I work with practices I

always send out a survey to the team members and the feedback that I get more often than not is that their opinions don't seem to count. This is, of course, your practice and you, rightfully so, have final say on everything. But the team needs to know and feel that their opinions are valued as well. I'll demonstrate the fairness issue by telling a story. One of my clients decided that he would pay for one of his assistants and her three children to fly to California to visit her mother because she didn't have the money for the trip. He assumed that she would keep this a secret but the secret was evidently too big for her to keep and the other assistant got wind of what had happened. Can you imagine how she felt when she found out? Disappointed. Hurt. Unappreciated. The dentist did try to make things right by giving her a bonus but too much damage had been done and she later handed in her notice.

3. *Sympathetic Help on Personal Problems*: I have a very successful client in rural Mississippi who has been with me for many years. His family is right up there with his religion in being the most important two things in his life. Every member of his team knows that he expects their families to come before their jobs and, if ever they need time to take care of things at home, he will make sure they get it. You might think that people would take advantage of him but the reverse is actually true. They have such a high level of respect for him that they wouldn't ever consider taking advantage of him and if he ever needs a little extra from them, they will willingly give it to him.

4. *Job Security*: Many people, if not most, who work in a dental practice live paycheck to paycheck. They can't afford to have hours cut back or to be laid off. They have to know that they have job security. So, when a boss comes swooping in like a seagull

threatening to cut hours or get rid of people if they all don't make sure the practice produces more, his actions have the exact opposite effect. What he needs instead is to get the team committed and energized towards solving the problem rather than threatening them. It's likely that if this scenario took place at all there would be many things wrong in the practice and leadership is probably one of them.

5. *Good Wages*: As I said before, as long as the BAM is met, wages fall to number five in the ranking. It has to be taken out of the equation by making sure they are paid fairly and, I would add, a little bit above average for the area. This is just good practice. Don't hesitate to do little things for them like pay for their lunches if you have a staff meeting during the lunch hour and, of course, pay them for their time. Pay for their time during continuing education if you mandate it. These expenses amount to a fraction of your overhead and the last thing that you want is for them to feel like you are nickel and diming them and begrudge spending anything extra on them.

6. *Interesting Work*: Everybody's job consists of mundane tasks we would rather not do, tasks that get relegated to the bottom of the pile. Wouldn't life be just lovely if our jobs consisted only of fun, interesting work? There is something that bosses can do to make our jobs more interesting and that is to identify people's strengths and weaknesses and to capitalize on their strengths by giving them work they love to do while working around their weaknesses. Markus Buckingham wrote several books on this subject that would make interesting reading namely, *First Break All the Rules* and *Now Discover Your Strengths*. Another factor is to embrace continuing education. Everybody loves to learn new

skills and, if you have anybody on your team who doesn't, they should probably seek their employment happiness elsewhere.

7. *Promotion/Growth Opportunities*: I bet that, when you read this, you thought that this surely wasn't possible in a dental practice. There are many areas of promotion possible within each individual department in dentistry such as: expanded functions assistant, lead assistant, lead hygienist, OSHA officer, HIPAA officer, office manager, marketing manager, to name just a few. Once you've started developing leaders throughout the team you can assign more responsibility and accountability which, in turn, allows you more time to do what you do best which is practice dentistry. You become a macro manager instead of a micro manager and your administrative and staff headaches and time are significantly reduced.

8. *Personal Loyalty to Workers*: Your entire team should be focused not only on teamwork and being willing to help one another out without question, but also focused on setting one another up for success. This means that everyone does their job to the very best of their ability to that nobody else has to pick up the pieces or correct others' mistakes. This means that the team knows that you will back them up and support their decisions within reason, of course. This encourages them to use their initiative and do what's right for the patient without having to run everything through their boss.

9. *Good Working Conditions*: There is plenty that falls under this category. An attractive office that they can be proud of is one. The technology they need to perform their jobs efficiently and effectively. Good hours. Good perks. Occasional social get-togethers. Little things on occasion like a Starbucks run, lunches, birthday cards, hire date anniversary, Christmas

party, Bath and Body Works basket (for everyone), and even sometimes a $50 gift card for a job well done or an exceptional month. These are all things that need to be planned out ahead of time, scheduled and incorporated into the year or else, believe me, they won't happen.

10. *Tactful Discipline:* By now I hope everybody knows to praise in public and discipline in private. It is equally important to separate the problem from the person. It isn't a bad person that did something but rather a person who did something badly. Remember that it's always a good idea to sandwich criticism between what's going well.

Getting the team on board, dialed in and committed to you, your vision and your practice is the cornerstone for creating an Above and Beyond practice. Treat your team right and they will, in turn, treat your patients right. Treat your team right and they will give you their loyalty and their willingness to give you their utmost effort. Treat your team right and everything else will succeed.

Worth Quoting

"It is not the employer who pays the wages. Employers only handle the money. It is the customer who pays the wages."

Henry Ford

Patient Loyalty

So now that we've got the team committed and on board and willing to help lead the charge, let's look at how to create this incredible Above and Beyond experience for our patients. Developing such
a practice is not about doing a 180 and it's not about taking your
practice from where you are to outstanding. *Rather, it's about **consistently** doing everything you do 5% to 10% better than your competition.*
That means every single time. If you can't do it every single time,
don't do it at all because there's nothing worse than setting high
expectations one visit only to have those expectations dashed the
next. In addition, you want to do a handful of things that, when it
happens to your patients, they say, "Wow!" These should be things
that are easily woven into the day-to-day operation of the practice
so that they can be done seamlessly. At Disney they say that they
"over manage" every aspect of the guest experience -- every single
step of the guest experience is spelled out clearly and specifically
for their cast members to follow. There is no ambiguity and everybody does it the same way with the same level of enthusiasm so
that when you have a Disney experience, it feels completely natural.

My husband and I were at a Disney Institute three-and-a-half-day
Leadership Excellence course. On the last night we had reservations
to have dinner at one of the restaurants at our resort. We were about
thirty minutes early and asked whether we could be seated. They
told us it wouldn't be a problem and asked us to wait in a small
alcove where several other couples were already waiting. Our hostess
walked directly up to us (even though there were several other people
waiting) and asked us to accompany her to the table. "Ah-Ha!" said
my little brain, "I wonder how they just did that." When I asked,
the hostess confided that the person at the desk always wrote some

distinguishing feature about the person/s she was to escort to their table and, as it happened, I was wearing a bright red jacket making it simple to identify who I was without ever having seen me before. If Disney can do it, so can your dental practice team. There is no longer any excuse for anybody not to walk right up to the person in the waiting room with confidence even if they have never met them.

Worth Quoting

"You'll never have a product or price advantage again. They can be easily duplicated, but a strong customer service culture can't be copied."

Jerry Fritz

Meet your Patients Where *They* Are

One of the key ingredients to really caring about your patients and getting case acceptance is to meet them where they are instead of trying to impose your vision on them. Having perfect teeth may be your vision but it may not be theirs. Sometimes it can be very difficult not to want them to have the same expectations as you do and to be able to understand why they don't. It's your job to find out where they are, meet them there, and then begin the process of bringing them along. The process may be a long one, it may take months or even years, and they may never reach *your* level of satisfaction. Your job is to *listen* and to develop a relationship of trust and bring them as far along as you can no matter how long it takes. If you can do this one thing for each of your patients you will already be ahead of 90 percent of dental practices out there. This is a skill to be cultivated and nurtured. The best source I know of to learn this is from Dr. Paul Homoly and his book and videos on *Getting Patients To Say "Yes" to Treatment.*

Worth Quoting

"Quality in a service or product is not what you put into it.
It is what the client or customer gets out of it."

Peter Drucker

Creating "Wow" Moments

Earlier in this chapter we discussed creating a handful of "wow" moments for your patients. You and your team need to decide what works best for you and what has the greatest positive impact on patients. It has to be something that isn't difficult to implement or it's a fairly sure bet that it either won't be done consistently or won't be done at all. As with everything else, whatever you do should be clearly outlined step by step so that everyone has a specific blueprint for their individual roles and responsibilities in the process. Try to do things that involve most, if not all, of your patients most, if not all, of the time. Here are just a few examples of what my clients have done, but you and your team can get really creative and come up with some fabulous ideas:

- *Beverage bar:* The best ones that I have seen have a mini fridge with assorted soft drinks, juice and water, a coffee maker such as a Keurig, and often something to eat such as biscotti and some apples.
- *Chairside Comfort:* Several of my practices have a heated vibrating chair such as a HoMedics pad that can be covered for ease of sterilization. They offer heated neck pillows and warm damp towels.
- *Heated Loo Seat:* Don't roll your eyes at this one. It was an idea from one of my most productive clients ever – a heated toilet seat. It costs less than $100 and my client swore that it was the most commented upon thing he ever did for his patients. He also paid really close attention to transforming his patients' bathroom from something cold and sterile into a warm, cozy, inviting place.

Connecting

Connect with your patients. No, I mean, *really connect*. Honor them with your undivided attention when you're communicating with them. When you're speaking with them, stop what you're doing, pay attention, listen and maintain eye contact. And, in addition, pay attention to their body language, tone, and pace.

There are a couple of things to remember here: 55 percent of everything we perceive in communication comes from body language, 38 percent from tone and pace, and only 7 percent from the actual words spoken. While the words we speak are very important, the greatest impact we have during our interactions with others comes from body language and tone and pace. One of the most common shortcomings I see is a dental team member or doctor conducting a critical discussion with the patient without any eye contact because the patient is lying down or looking in the opposite direction. Whenever there is a case to be presented, financial arrangement to be made, or treatment to be discussed, dental professionals need to make sure the patient is sitting up and the team member or doctor are seated at the same eye-level as the patient, facing them, and with masks removed.

Verbal skills need to be personalized so that they feel comfortable for the team member delivering them. Change them to suit you, while still keeping the message the same. Here are some suggestions but feel free to add to them as you proceed.

- When either the hygienist or assistant go out to the reception room to invite the patient back, never stand in the doorway but rather go right out into the reception room and invite them to accompany you back into the clinical area: "Fred, it's good to see you again; please come in," or, "Hi Fred, my name is Nancy and I'm Dr. Smith's hygienist. I'll take care of you from here. Please come in." Remember that the patient probably feels relatively safe in the reception room but the clinical area is another thing; it is filled with strange smells and sounds and nasty needles and drills that hurt.
- Let the patient walk in front of you if possible: "Fred, it will be the second room on the right."

- When the patient is seated and *before* you lay the chair back, sit facing the patient at the same eye level and ask: "Today we're going to do those three fillings on the lower left. What questions do you have before we get started?"

- When the doctor enters the treatment room, tell him or her all the information that you have for example: Periodontal status, recommended interval between hygiene appointments, restorative concerns, and patient concerns.

- Ideally, doctors will sit at the same eye level as the patients, masks removed, relaxed and facing the patient as they introduce themselves.

- A typical hand-off from the hygienist may go as follows: "Doctor, Fred is doing a good job with his home-care. We still have a few 4 mm pockets in the posterior areas so I have recommended that he remain on a 3-month interval to prevent any back-sliding. Fred is having sensitivity with that tooth on the upper right at the back, number 15. I have an intraoral picture on the screen; there is a large silver filling on that tooth and we have discussed the possibility of a crown."

- Remember to ask open-ended questions: "Fred, what questions do you have?" instead of: "Fred, do you have any questions?" Open-ended questions are defined as those that cannot be answered with a simple "yes" or "no."

- The clinical team should make sure that the patient has clearly understood and summarize the next appointment/s: "Did everything that Dr. Smith say make sense to you? Great. I'm going to take you up to Suzie at the front desk and we need to schedule you for two appointments. One is to do the fillings on the lower left side and the other is to see our hygienist for your periodontal cleaning."

- When bringing the patient up to the front desk the clinical team reiterates what was done today and what needs to be scheduled for next: "Suzie, today we finished the fillings on the upper arch and Fred needs two further appointments. One is for those three fillings on the lower left, that should take Doctor about forty minutes, and the other is for a periodontal cleaning appointment. Fred, you were a great patient today and we look forward to seeing you next time."

Worth Quoting

"Spend a lot of time talking to customers face to face. You'd be amazed how many companies don't listen to their customers."

Ross Perot

Appointment Wrap-Ups

I literally cringe when I listen to many assistants and hygienists as they get the patient ready to dismiss to the front desk. Usually they are taking off the bib, gathering the chart and routing sheet and, all the while, talking to the patient. Guess where their focus is? Right, it's on getting the patient out of the chair instead of focusing on them and making sure all their questions have been answered and they have a clear understanding of what was done today and what needs to be scheduled for next. At the end of the appointment, once the dentist has left the treatment room, the hygienist or assistant should wrap-up and summarize treatment done today as well as the next appointment that needs to be scheduled. Remember that during an interaction, 55% of what is perceived comes from body language. This is why body positioning is extremely important. The assistant or hygienist should sit facing the patient at or slightly below eye level with a relaxed posture. They should take a big breath (which also helps with relaxation) and ask: "Fred, what questions do you have about the treatment that Doctor recommended?" (Notice the open-ended question.) Follow this with, "Today we did the initial crown prep on the tooth on the lower left. In two weeks time we will need to place the permanent crown. That will be about a forty minute appointment and we'll have Suzie schedule that when I take you up to the front desk. As Doctor mentioned, you're past due for your cleaning so we'll also ask Suzie to schedule that appointment at the same time. Fred, what questions do you have before I take you up to the front?"

When the dental assistant brings the patient back to the front desk, they should not merely hand off the chart and be off. But a better method is to take the time to again reinforce what you've done and what the next treatment will be. Have a brief three-way conversation between yourself, the patient, and the receptionist that establishes the future actions to be taken. Continue to be warm and make eye contact with the patient. Ask the receptionist to schedule an appointment for whatever future treatment, which will naturally set her up to offer the patient a choice of several possible dates. By working together, you both reassure the patient and make it very easy to book future appointments.

Establishing Value for the Hygiene Appointment

The majority of cancellations and broken appointments occur in the hygiene schedule. Patients are usually scheduled for their next appointment at the end of their last appointment, which means that they have 3-6 months to forget about it. There are several different strategies that can help establish greater value for the hygiene appointment and thereby prevent the high rate of missed appointments.

Get everyone talking "hygiene" to the patient. Studies show that people need to hear something seven times before it becomes set in their memories. More often than not, when restorative patients who do not have their next hygiene appointment scheduled are brought up to the front desk, they are reminded that they need to reschedule their hygiene appointment. This is usually done as an afterthought thereby losing much of its value and significance.

A better way is, immediately upon seating the patient, for the assistant to remind them that it has been a while since their last hygiene appointment and the doctor will take a look and see how they are doing. Don't minimize the importance of the hygiene appointment by saying things such as "just a cleaning," or "a little bit of bleeding."

When the doctor enters the treatment room the assistant will alert the doctor who is then able to reinforce the importance of scheduling their next hygiene appointment. Doctors stress the importance of scheduling the next hygiene visit during the hygiene exam and why the recommended interval is so important. Be sure to focus on the benefit the patient will receive from getting back on a regular hygiene schedule.

Before the assistant takes the patient up to the front desk she will inform the patient of the appointment/s that need to be scheduled. During the handoff at the front desk the assistant will inform the scheduler of the appointment that needs to be scheduled and then finally the scheduler will hand the patient the appointment card and reiterate the date and time of the appointment. This makes a grand total of six times the patient has heard about the importance of scheduling thereby almost guaranteeing that they will remember and keep their appointment time.

Post-op Calls

Yup, this really is still number one when it comes to public relations and has a *major impact* on your patients. This is the single most important thing a doctor can do to make his/her patients feel really special. Sometimes these calls are delegated to another staff member but, beware, they lose about 90% of their effectiveness and impact when not done by the doctor.

Some guidelines to follow are that the calls should be made at the end of the day before the doctor goes home or from a mobile phone on the way home. Most of the calls will go to voicemail and it's very rare that a patient keeps you talking even if you reach them. Doctors should call at least 50 percent of their patients. Preferably everyone who receives anesthetic will be called and this includes the hygienist calling their scaling and root planing patients.

Keep the verbiage simple: "Fred, this is Dr. Smith calling, I'm calling to check in with you to make sure you're feeling comfortable after your procedure today, (pause—wait for a response). Great. Fred thanks for coming in, we really appreciate patients like you/it was great meeting you today/we look forward to seeing you next time."

Notes to Patients

This is another must-do item. It makes the patients feel special and it keeps you on the forefront of their minds. Don't forget to use a really nice card not some cheapo version you got at the Dollar Store.

There are many occasions to send out cards to patients such as thank you for the referral, for patiently waiting while we saw an emergency, for completing treatment, welcome to the practice, for becoming a new patient, for making our day, for being a great patient, weddings, graduations, sympathy, and so forth. While you won't want to send cards for all occasions, decide exactly what occasions you will send cards for and then do it, you've guessed it — every single time.

In the case where the doctor may want to write a personal note, prepare the card along with a stamped envelope and place it on the doctor's desk.

In some cases you may want to include a gift card to Starbucks or something similar.

Except in cases such as sympathy cards, it is always a good idea to enclose a couple of business cards along with a handwritten P.S.

stating that you really appreciate the referral of their friends and co-workers.

Sample verbiage for a thank you for the referral: "You really made our day! Fred came in today based on your recommendation. Thanks for the trust you have placed in us, we truly value each and every referral. It is a pleasure having you as a patient. Thank you so much.

Sample verbiage when a patient is kept waiting: I just want to thank you again for waiting so patiently while we treated an emergency on Wednesday. I know your time is precious and I appreciate your flexibility. It is a pleasure having you as a patient. Thank you so much.

New Patient Calls

Before you dismiss this idea as one that would never fly in your practice, one of the highest producing dentists in Colorado Springs does this and he gets almost 100 new patients a month, most of them from patient referrals. He calls his new patients two days before their appointment to welcome them into the practice. He says: "Fred, this is Dr. Smith and I see you are scheduled to visit our dental practice on Thursday at 3:00 p.m. I just want to welcome you and to ask if there is anything I need to know to make your visit more comfortable?" What this doctor achieves is the patients show up more often for their appointment, they definitely get the WOW factor, they accept more treatment plans, keep their ensuing appointments, and pay their bills!

Above and Beyond Action Items

The key to patient loyalty is actually team loyalty. Get your team excited to help make patients happy.

- Look at the list of employee "needs" and make efforts to improve the areas that matter most to them, *not* to you.
- Patient loyalty is a matter of *consistently* doing everything just 5-10 percent better than your competition. Small steps can be taken to get there.
- Meet your patients where they are by listening and developing trust so you can establish a treatment plan that they will be ready to accept.
- Create "Wow!" moments – choose a few things you can do consistently that will impress your patients and make them feel at home.
- Connect with patients on a personal level by sitting at eye level and honoring them with your undivided attention.
- Establish the value of future appointments and reinforce this throughout the visit, right up to the check out.

- Doctors should make brief post-op calls to patients, particularly any that had anesthesia. This has a major impact for patients with minimal effort for you.
- Notes to patients are a must-do item. Choose which occasions you will send a note for (e.g., referrals, birthdays, sympathy, etc.) and do it *every time.*
- New patient calls allow the doctor to start to build patient trust and connections before they even arrive in the office.

CHAPTER 6

THE FOURTH LINK: INCREASED PROFITABILITY

If everyone is moving forward together, then success takes care of itself.
– Henry Ford

This is one of my favorite quotes and it really encapsulates the core message of my consulting work. When a team moves together towards a common goal, one that is focused on creating the best possible environment not only for their patients but for themselves as well, the result is loyal patients who return and refer, and ultimately, greater profitability, even when profitability was not the main goal initially.

When people ask me what the greatest predictors of successful leaders are, I say "Clarity!" If you are clear about your direction, if you articulate it to your team simply and succinctly, if you provide a step-by-step roadmap for your team to follow, they will gladly get on board with you. They will *want* to join with you and carry your vision forward. Clarity breeds passion within a team because they know where they're going and they know how to get there. Clarity gives meaning to the work they do. They understand how their jobs contribute towards the big picture. There's a certain synergy created by clarity within a team. People give more than they usually would on their own by themselves.

This is why when you organize the operation, it's so important to outline the steps along the way towards reaching your goal. And, don't worry—you do not have to come up with all the answers because the more the team is involved in the process the better.

Worth Quoting

"Organizing is what you do before you do something,
so that when you do it, it is not all mixed up."

A.A Milne, author of *Winnie the Pooh*

Organizing the Operation

When organizing any systems, policies or procedures within your practice, there are, of course, some vital management and communications systems that need to be in place, such as the organizational hierarchy, position descriptions, and communication channels, like morning meetings or huddles, staff meetings, planning meetings, and gathering and tracking data to monitor your financial progress.

I believe that every aspect of the patient experience should be *over-managed*. By that I mean recording the minutest detail as part of the job descriptions and expectations. Expand upon the detail you might normally provide. Instead of merely saying, "greet the patient," consider this: "Look up when the patient enters the reception room, make eye contact and smile, stand up, shake their hand and greet them by name using one of the following verbal skills depending on the patient and situation..." See how much more detail there is with this set of instructions? Each aspect should be spelled out to provide absolute clarity. People want to know the steps so that they can follow them with confidence, knowing that they are doing what is expected of them.

And, of course, everything you design should be viewed through the lens of whether or not this helps move you closer to your vision.

The following steps can, and usually *should,* be done with input from the relevant team members. Any time you can involve team members in the decision-making process they naturally feel a greater sense of ownership and, in turn, they will put their collective shoulder to the wheel to make sure it is implemented. In fact, sometimes the most successful outcomes take place when the team is given the problem and allowed to come up with the best solution on their own, thereby guaranteeing buy-in from all concerned.

1. Envision the Goal

One of the most common mistakes made by leaders and managers alike is to try to improve the current situation when systems are not running smoothly. If something is not working as well as it should, they try to come up with incremental steps for improvement. On the surface this may sound like a good strategy, but it is counter productive in one key respect; while it may *improve* the situation, because you're not starting with the ideal scenario in mind, it is very possible that you will settle for something far less than the ideal. It is really important to view things from the perspective of how this would look, feel, and sound if it were being done *perfectly*. To coin a phrase from Disney, strive for perfection and settle for excellence.

From the vantage point of perfection, you can move forward towards reaching this goal by determining where the gaps lie between the current situation and the ultimate goal.

2. Determine the Gaps

Now that you have the goal figured out, determine what needs to be done to help you reach it. Make sure to break the steps down into specific functions and tasks and look for ways in which to measure your progress. Look at the existing system with a critical eye. Just because something has always been done a certain way, doesn't mean that way belongs in the current strategy. Toss it out or change it if it isn't working.

3. Develop Policies and Procedures

There should be a structured process for the team to follow. Identify and make use of team members who are enthusiastic about the project. Again, if you have members of your team who are not, it may be time for them to seek their happiness elsewhere. I know this is a concept that is easy to understand but difficult to implement. I have a client in Michigan who had put up with a surly, unproductive office manager for seven years. Good morning, good night, please, and thank you were not a part of her vocabulary. He knew he should get rid of her but in all his 23 years in practice he had *never fired anyone.* When he discovered that she was stealing from him and finally made the decision to let her go, he told me that he didn't realize just how much he dreaded coming to work each day! It's often only when you get rid of a disgruntled team member that is poisoning the rest of the apple cart that you realize just how bad it was. You have an obligation to your business to have the best people on board and you have an obligation to your team members to provide a harmonious work environment.

- Adjust position descriptions if necessary.
- Provide clarity surrounding individual roles.
- Develop a detailed written policy for the team to follow.
- Continually work on refining the system. Make it the team's responsibility to develop solutions to inefficiencies and other problems.
- Train, train, train.

Worth Quoting

"An idea can only become a reality once it is broken down into organized, actionable elements."

Scott Belsky, *Making Ideas Happen: Overcoming the Obstacles Between Vision and Reality*

---

4. Accountability and Communication

Give the team members as much leeway as possible as long as the goals are being met. Your role is to stay as far away as you can from micro-managing and to view things at the macro level. There's nothing worse than a leader who is constantly micro-managing his or her team, which really takes the wind out of team members' sails. They begin to think, "Why bother, if he/she thinks they can do it all? What do they need my input and energy for?" I know this can be difficult especially for many dentists who are perfectionists and want everything to be done just so. It reminds me of the story of a client of mine who had a horrible time letting go and delegating to the team. He'd ask someone to do something for him and the next thing you know he'd done it himself. His team felt like he didn't trust them to do anything right and you could just feel the motivation literally drain out of them. We worked on this for quite a while, not just from his micromanagement perspective but also in helping the team realize that they needed to keep him informed of what was being done along the way. Now, six months later, my client feels like a giant weight has been lifted from his shoulders. And, yes, his team may not do things exactly like he would but they are perfectly willing and capable of reaching the end goal. Be prepared to step in if need be to provide guidance and clarity but only if you absolutely need to or if they ask you for your help.

Determine how you are going to monitor the results, who is responsible for tracking them, and when and where the results will be shared with the team. Determine how frequently the team will meet to discuss progress and determine if adjustments need to be made. Decide how incremental individual and collective successes will be acknowledged. Make sure the system for communication within the organization is established and effective for the specific venture.

Worth Quoting

"The most difficult thing is the organization of people and the expression of your intentions. It's very easy to have a picture in your head and to imagine that you've told everybody about what you need."

Neil Jordan

Team Support

Of course, you will want to get the very best out of your team in this process. According to a research study by Accor Services, 90 percent of leaders say employee engagement is critical. And yet, their study found that 75 percent of respondents have no system in place to motivate their employees. It is not surprising then that the same study found 42 percent of the global workforce says they are not motivated at work. A Gallup study of American workers puts that figure at 70 percent. This is no minor matter.

You developed the goal and organized the operation—now the focus shifts to motivating the team to do a good job. If you want to get the most out of your team, they must be engaged and excited to help you meet your goals. If they are not, there will be little incentive for them to work hard for you.

It is no big secret that an engaged and motivated team ultimately leads to greater profitability. But did you realize a disengaged team can actually cost you money? The same Gallup research study found that the top 25 percent of teams versus the bottom 25 percent in any workplace have nearly 50 percent fewer accidents and have 41 percent fewer quality defects. The study states: "What's more, teams in the top 25 percent versus the bottom 25 percent incur far less in healthcare costs. So having too few engaged employees means our workplaces are less safe, employees have more quality defects, and disengagement — which results from terrible managers — is driving up the country's healthcare costs."

In order to do the very best job possible and to get the job done, your team needs to feel empowered, to feel part of the process, to be challenged and to grow and they need the tools and resources to get the job done. Let's take a closer look at each of these aspects:

Empowerment

To assist with empowerment, individual roles and levels of authority need to be clarified at all levels. Determine who does what, where ultimate accountability and responsibilities lie and who reports to whom. Encourage the team to look for better ways of doing things—they may come up with something you never considered. As the leader, be open to the possibility of things being done somewhat differently than *you* would do. Allow creativity as long as the goal is being met and a good job is being done. Your team should be encouraged to make decisions and be held accountable for these decisions. Give the team as much leeway as possible but know when to get involved and when not to. Do not micromanage the process.

Collaboration

I have been touching upon this aspect throughout the book. Collaboration is key and studies show that effective teams are actually more satisfied in their jobs. To promote collaboration, make sure your team members know how they are contributing to the overall goal so they understand how their work benefits the team and the practice. Build employee input into your meeting agenda and respond accordingly. Train your team on effective communication strategies and create an environment that encourages open and honest communication. When working with practices, I love to see and openly encourage active debates where everybody has their say and feels like they have been heard even though not every suggestion or argument is incorporated into the overall picture. Differentiate employee issues into two categories: those that require action and those that require listening and guidance. Sometimes employees just want to feel heard.

Development

Most people will be dissatisfied if they feel like they are in a dead-end job with no hope of advancement. Even people who are not terribly career-oriented will appreciate growth and development in the workplace. Give your team access to training and coaching both from within the business and external options. Continuing education classes are an excellent opportunity for employees to expand their knowledge and skills.

Resources

This may seem obvious, but people need the right resources to do their jobs properly. Don't force people to make do—give your team members what they need to do their jobs. Take into account the concerns of your team and be willing to step in and make changes when necessary. Reward your team when they come up with creative and innovative ideas on how to use resources more wisely.

Worth Quoting

"Learn to handle the passing of time. It takes time to build a career; it takes time to make changes, so give your project time. Also give your people time; if you're working with people give them time to learn, grow, change, develop, and produce. And here is the big one--give yourself time. It takes time to master something new. It takes time to make changes and refinement in philosophy, as well as activity. Give yourself time to learn, time to get it, time to start some momentum, time to finally achieve. It is easy to be impatient with yourself."

Jim Rohn

Huddles

I've mentioned this in passing throughout the preceding chapters, but team huddles are an excellent tool that should be incorporated in every practice. The huddle is the most important team meeting of all. Not only does it help the team prepare for the day, it also serves to inspire and motivate the team. Independent studies consistently show that an effective huddle helps to increase production by an average of $100 to $200 per day, which is $20,000 to $40,000 a year for the average practice. So if you don't want to leave that kind of money on the table, here are some strategies for holding effective huddles:

Huddle Guidelines

Huddle Leader: I strongly believe that the huddle should be led by the team rather than the doctor. Rotating the lead amongst team members on a weekly basis will help promote accountability, leadership, and the interconnection of the entire team. Obviously the Doctor will be present and should participate whenever necessary.

The role of the huddle leader is simple. He or she ensures that the meeting starts and ends on time because sometimes teams tend to get bogged down discussing the details of one patient. The huddle leader's job is to keep the team on task and on time so that everything is covered. If necessary, a more in depth discussion can continue after the meeting.

It is a good idea for the huddle leader to bring a fun or inspirational quote for the end of the huddle. Teams often have a good time with this and it sets a positive tone for the rest of the day.

Preparation: One of the key elements to the success of a huddle lies in the preparation. Each team member should review, prepare, and make notes on their own patients, or the portion of the huddle they are to contribute to, before the huddle starts. When the individual team members find the time to do this is up to the practice or the individual. Some practices find it best to come in 10 minutes before the huddle while others prefer to prepare during the previous day.

The rule of thumb is that nobody should have to open a chart during the huddle because they will already have the pertinent information at their finger tips and should only to refer to a chart occasionally.

We recommend that charts are pulled (unless your practice is chartless), routing slips printed, and courtesy reminder calls are made by 11 a.m. the previous day. This gives everyone an adequate window of time in which to review their charts for the following day.

Running the huddle: Hold the huddle in a private area where patients are not able to overhear. Place a framed sign at the front desk stating that you are in a short meeting preparing for the day and will be with them shortly. It's a great idea to go the extra mile and place small bottles of water and or juice, and the morning newspaper next to the sign.

The huddle should take no longer than ten to fifteen minutes for a single doctor practice. The best time to hold the huddle is the first thing in the morning. Due to varied staff and practice schedules, this is not always possible and some practices have to find creative ways to solve this problem such as holding the huddle at the end of the day or in the first fifteen minutes of the lunch hour.

The flow of the huddle: The huddle is your snapshot in time between yesterday, today, and tomorrow. You will want to take a look back at yesterday to see what went right and what you don't want to repeat. This should only take a minute or two. You will want to take a look at tomorrow to see what's on the schedule and what actions, if any, need to be taken. Again, this should only take a moment. 80 percent to 90 percent of the time should be spent on today.

We recommend creating a Huddle Folder that the huddle leader will bring to the huddle. In it should be stored the following: a master copy of yesterday's schedule (showing how the day began, emergencies that came in and appointments missed or rescheduled), copies of today's and the next day's schedule and a copy of the Huddle Checklist (see below).

Here is a sample of how a typical huddle should go:

Yesterday

The huddle leader distributes copies of yesterday's schedule and invites comments on what went right, what could be improved, and highlights the patients who did not schedule their next appointment.

Assistants/Hygienists Review Their Day

The huddle leader asks each of the assistant(s) and hygienist(s) in turn to review their day. They should each discuss the following items, much of which is available from the routing sheet:

Scheduled treatment: While it is redundant to discuss each line item as it is written on the schedule (e.g. Prophy, four bitewings, exam), there may be additional information regarding today's treatment that needs to be discussed (e.g. different type of anesthetic needed, patient has a gag reflex). In many cases, there will not be additional discussion points for each patient.

Does anyone need updated x-rays? Not only for bitewing x-rays but also for updating of full mouth series or panorex according to your practice's x-ray policy.

Does the patient have their next hygiene appointment scheduled: Obviously this one is just for restorative patients. Many people tell us that they always schedule patients for their next hygiene appointment when they check them out, which is great. However, we feel that it is important to know before the patient arrives so that it can be discussed in a manner that leaves no doubt in the patients' mind as to the importance of the appointment. The assistant should discuss it immediately upon seating the patient, alert the doctor when he or she comes in, the doctor should stress the importance, as does the assistant before taking the patient up to the front desk to check out, speak to the scheduling coordinator as the patient is handed off at the front desk and finally the scheduling coordinator confirms what the appointment is for, the date and time as the appointment card is handed to the patient. This makes a total of six times. Not only will it seem important to the patient but he or she will be much more likely to keep the appointment because of that. The appointment simply doesn't seem as important when casually mentioned during checkout at the front desk. To the patient it seems like an afterthought, something that really isn't that important anyway thereby resulting in more broken appointments.

Are there any family members that need an appointment? This can be obtained from the routing sheet. If a parent is scheduled, what better time to schedule a child who may be in need of an appointment?

Is there delayed or unappointed treatment? This is especially important in hygiene so that the hygienist can take intraoral pictures in preparation for the doctors' examination. It will also help the practice to recover from unexpected openings in the schedule.

Nitrous oxide patients: This information helps the practice to be prepared for the patients' visit.

Are lab cases in for today and tomorrow? Make sure you know the status of lab cases for the next two days' patients.

Did the doctor and hygienist make post-op calls the previous evening? Post-op calls remain the most important public relations thing a practice can do. We recommend that hygienists call all of their scaling and root planing patients and the doctor call all patients who received anesthetic. We also recommend that the calls be made in the evening before leaving or on the way home. While an assistant making the calls is better than no call at all, it is an excellent practice when the doctor makes the calls personally.

Administrators Review the Following

The huddle leader then turns to the administrators for information on the following:

New patient information: Such as who referred the patient to the practice, areas of concern, when the patient last saw a dentist, whether x-rays have been forwarded and so forth.

Pre-Med patients: Confirm that pre-medication has been called in for all pre-med patients.

Openings for today: State where in the schedule there are openings today.

Emergency time for today: If you have a full schedule, it is helpful to identify a time in the morning and the afternoon where an emergency patient can be scheduled.

Birthday, family news, and TLC patients: Share any pertinent information regarding today's patients.

Financial information on today's patients: For example, what financial arrangements have been made for treatment? Are there past due balances that need to be collected or is there insurance information that needs to be gathered?

Tomorrow

The huddle leader then reviews the following day and invites comments from the team. Typically, the main issues are:

- Are there openings in tomorrow's schedule? This enables the entire team to proactively search for ways in which to fill these openings.
- Is the practice scheduled to production? A proactive approach will help the practice to reach their goals.

Looking at the following day's schedule with a critical eye is important. The team may be able to uncover issues such as patients that may benefit from an extra courtesy reminder call or additional treatment that could be completed on a patient.

Quote For the Day

The huddle leader then shares his or her quote for the day and adjourns the meeting.

Huddle Checklist

Huddle leader brings the following:
- Copies of yesterday's schedule
- Copies of today's schedule
- Copies of tomorrow's schedule

Yesterday:
Review the good points and what could be improved on yesterday's schedule

Today:
Assistants/Hygienists review the following:
- Scheduled treatment
- Does anyone need updated x-rays
- Does the patient have their next hygiene appointment scheduled
- Are there any family members in need of an appointment
- Is there delayed or unappointed treatment
- Nitrous oxide patients
- Are lab cases in for today and tomorrow
- Did the doctor and hygienists make their post-op calls

Administrators review the following:
- New patient information
- Pre-med patients
- Openings for today

- Emergency time for today
- Birthday, family news and TLC patients
- Financial information on today's patients

Tomorrow:
- Are there any openings for tomorrow
- Is the practice scheduled to production

Quote for the day

Staff Meetings

Staff meetings are also vitally important to the success of any team. As a consultant, I see a direct correlation between organizational effectiveness and regular staff meetings. Holding staff meetings is one of the most effective things a practice can do to increase productivity, profitability and, most importantly, communication.

Staff Meeting Guidelines

Weekly Meeting Schedules: staff meetings should be at least thirty minutes long, however, once a month, usually the first meeting of the month, you should have a longer staff meeting. The longer meeting allows you to review the statistics for the previous month. Most of our teams are willing to hold the 30-minute staff meetings during the second half of lunch time. It is, of course, paid time for the team members. We recommend that you finish lunch before you begin your meeting so that everyone can focus. Paying attention while dishing and eating food creates an unwelcome distraction for everyone. This also means scheduling appointment(s) immediately before lunch time very carefully to avoid procedures that are likely to run over. Block your staff meetings into the schedule for six months in advance.

Meeting Binder: Start a "Meeting Binder," a three-ring binder with the following tabs: TAPs (Team Action Plans), Blank TAPs, and Agenda. Keep a TAP sheet for all your meetings—not just staff meetings. Any time two or more people meet, a TAP sheet should be filled out for future follow-up.

Blank Agenda Sheet: Post a blank Agenda sheet in a convenient place where everyone has access to it during the week so any team member has the opportunity to write down any items for discussion at the meeting. Keep in mind that the meeting is a group event and, therefore, if anything needs to be discussed between individuals, it probably does not belong in the staff meeting format but rather in a private discussion.

TAP sheet: "TAP," or Team Action Plan, is a sheet of one or more pages used to resolve a common complaint – much discussion but little or no action. Without the TAP, many excellent ideas are discussed but due to inaction, the same items resurface time and time again at staff meetings, a waste of everyone's time. By using a TAP sheet during the meeting, any decisions the team reaches on items for discussion are recorded on the current week's sheet. This TAP sheet is filed in the Meeting Binder and a copy is posted next to the Blank Agenda Sheet as a reminder to the team. One of the first things discussed at the next staff meeting is the status of the previous week's TAPs and, anything that has not been completed is brought forward to the current week's TAP sheet.

Success Stories: It's a good idea to start the meeting on a positive note with individual success stories such as treatment that went well, patients who complimented you, or a team member who went above and beyond.

Staff Meeting Leader: Staff meetings are usually lead (facilitated) by the Doctor or the office manager. The meeting leader's role is to prepare for the meeting by bringing the Meeting Binder (which will have a copy of previous TAP sheets) and the Agenda Sheet. Be sure to start the meeting on time, end on time, and keep things moving along during the meeting so that everything can be addressed. Redirect if things get off track.

The leader should encourage participation. Use phrases like, "I'd like to hear everyone's views on this. Can we go round the room and have each person state their views in turn?" Another technique is to have everyone write down their thoughts in a three to four minute quiet time first and then solicit their comments. Keep in mind that you should maintain an environment of trust, respect and safety. Focus the group on expressing themselves in objective terms. For example, "Sara, I can see you're really upset about this, but let's focus today on the problem itself, not the people involved."

Assign someone to write up the TAP sheet during the meeting, file it in the Meeting Binder and post a copy along with a new Blank Agenda Sheet in the place that you have designated.

Rules of Engagement: Agree on the ground rules for the meeting as a group.

Examples are:

- Start and end the meeting on time.
- Follow your written agenda format.
- Only one person should speak at a time.
- Respect the leader or meeting facilitator.
- Create an environment of safety, respect and trust.
- Avoid finger pointing and put-downs.
- Problem-solve issues by defining clearly and objectively what is happening, what you want to have happen and possible solutions.
- At the closing of each topic, call for decisions and ask the person recording the TAP sheet to restate the assignments.

Staff Meeting Agenda

Bring the following items to the meeting:
- Meeting Binder with previous TAP sheets
- Most recent Weekly Monitor or Monthly Graphs
- Posted Agenda Sheet

Agenda:
- Share success stories from the week
- Review the most recent Weekly Monitor (or Monthly Graphs if this is the extended one-hour meeting)
- Discuss items for discussion from the Agenda Sheet that was posted and update your TAP sheet

---

> • Discuss the status of the previous TAP sheet and bring forward any uncompleted TAPs.
>
> *Adjourn the meeting*

Commit to the Results

Creating lasting change requires a commitment and ongoing support from the leader. In the beginning of the process of change, there is frequently an initial dip in productivity as the team adjusts to the change. As it begins to take root and the team begins to embrace it, the trend reverses and the upswing begins. Once the desired goal is reached, many leaders assume incorrectly that the team will continue to implement the changes ad infinitum.

Sadly, this is not the case. After the initial thrill of reaching the goal is over, there is a natural downward drift towards the previous status quo. This is the critical period where the leader needs to step in and lend his/her support. This is the time when the effort needs to be bolstered with key repeatable messages reminding everyone of the goal. Put posters stating the goal on the walls, discuss it during staff meetings, morning meetings, or huddles, and liberally give individual praise and encouragement. This allows time for the changes to become lasting until they ultimately form part of the culture of the organization.

Say, for example, you own a dental practice and your goal for your team is to proactively build relationships with each other and your patients. There's a big difference between doing this proactively versus reactively. Being reactive means that you are friendly in response to someone else. A proactive approach means you initiate friendliness, empathy, active listening, and sharing. You can see how a major cultural shift like this will take time to take hold.

Worth Quoting

"First comes thought; then organization of that thought, into ideas and plans; then transformation of those plans into reality. The beginning, as you will observe, is in your imagination."

Napoleon Hill

There are four strategies for ensuring the goal is not only reached but is sustained into the future.

1. Establishing the goal

Work alongside the team to encourage raising the bar and continuing to improve. Divide long-term or overarching goals into more manageable mini goals. Establish your goals for attention to detail, efficiency, customer service, and safety since these play a measurable part in improving bottom-line results and will set your practice apart from all others in the community.

For example, if your overarching goal is to achieve patient loyalty, one mini goal could be to implement some amazing patient experience that leaves the patients saying, "Wow, now *that's* cool". Make sure this is communicated to the team and that they understand the steps involved in making that happen. *You* need to make it important; if you make it important to you, it will in turn be important to the team.

2. *Quantify, monitor, and communicate results*

Keep your measures simple by only measuring what is important. Encourage the team to take ownership of these measurable results. Inform your team of the results. It's a bit like playing sports, if nobody tells you the score, you don't know if you're winning or not.

In the last chapter, we discussed the many monitors you will be using to track your business and by extension, patient satisfaction, and loyalty. There are many components involved and as a business owner, they are useful and important to you. I have had many dentists I work with tell me that they share these monitor graphs with their teams and they were disappointed because they felt like the team did not care. "I stopped giving it to them because their eyes just glazed over as they flipped through them. What's the point?"

Remember that there is a big difference between you, the business owner, and your team. The old adage that less is more really holds true here. It isn't that your team doesn't care but they may be overwhelmed with information if you hand them twenty charts and graphs, the majority of which don't even relate to their jobs.

Figure out the best two or three monitors that are most important to the team and only distribute those. Since there are just a
couple highlighted, the team members can process and understand
the information they need to know. You should be sure you are
quantifying the right things and that you are pinpointed and not
too broad. Customer Satisfaction, Missed Appointment, and New
Patient monitors might be useful to office staff. Case acceptance,
Periodontal Ratios and Tray Setup Accuracy might be useful to the
hygienists and clinical assistants.

To go back to the example above, if you choose to distribute the
Reappointment and Missed Appointment Monitor, the team can
clearly see if their efforts at lowering the broken appointments are
paying off or if they need to take additional steps.

3. Recognize progress and provide feedback

Catch your team "doing things right." Give individual praise and
tie it to a specific result or action you have observed. Be clear
about your expectations. Have one-on-one meetings where you
link feedback and appreciation back to the goals and organizational values.

4. Stay the course

Be prepared for resistance and problems. Instead of changing course,
remain focused on the goal. Seek counsel from trusted colleagues
and advisors who have faced similar situations. Celebrate incremental successes. Things will not always be perfect as you work towards
your goal.

Above and Beyond Action Items

You must see the ultimate goal before you can create the ideal system.

- Envision your goal – try to decide what would be the perfect vision of your practice and team.
- Determine the gaps – don't try to fix a broken system but figure out what is missing that will get you to the ultimate goal.
- Develop policies and procedures for your team to follow. Remember that clarity is key here – adjustments to policies or roles should be in writing and communicated clearly.
- Get out of your own way – let your team have the freedom to do their jobs well, even if it isn't exactly how you might do it. As long as the overall goals are being met, you should not be micro-managing tasks.
- Decide how to monitor results and keep communication open with the team.
- Motivate your team so they are excited to reach the vision with you. Use empowerment, collaboration, development, and resources to achieve this.

- Incorporate huddles and staff meetings into your practice – these not only motivate staff but increase productivity.
- Commit to your goals and help your team to continue to raise the bar to get to the end result. Provide feedback and be sure to always recognize and reward progress.

SECTION III

How to Guarantee an Unbreakable Chain

An unbreakable chain starts with making the decision that you will do whatever it takes to go Above and Beyond. Be resolved as you decide where to go and how to get there. Make sure your team is motivated and engaged so that they will be excited to get to that goal.

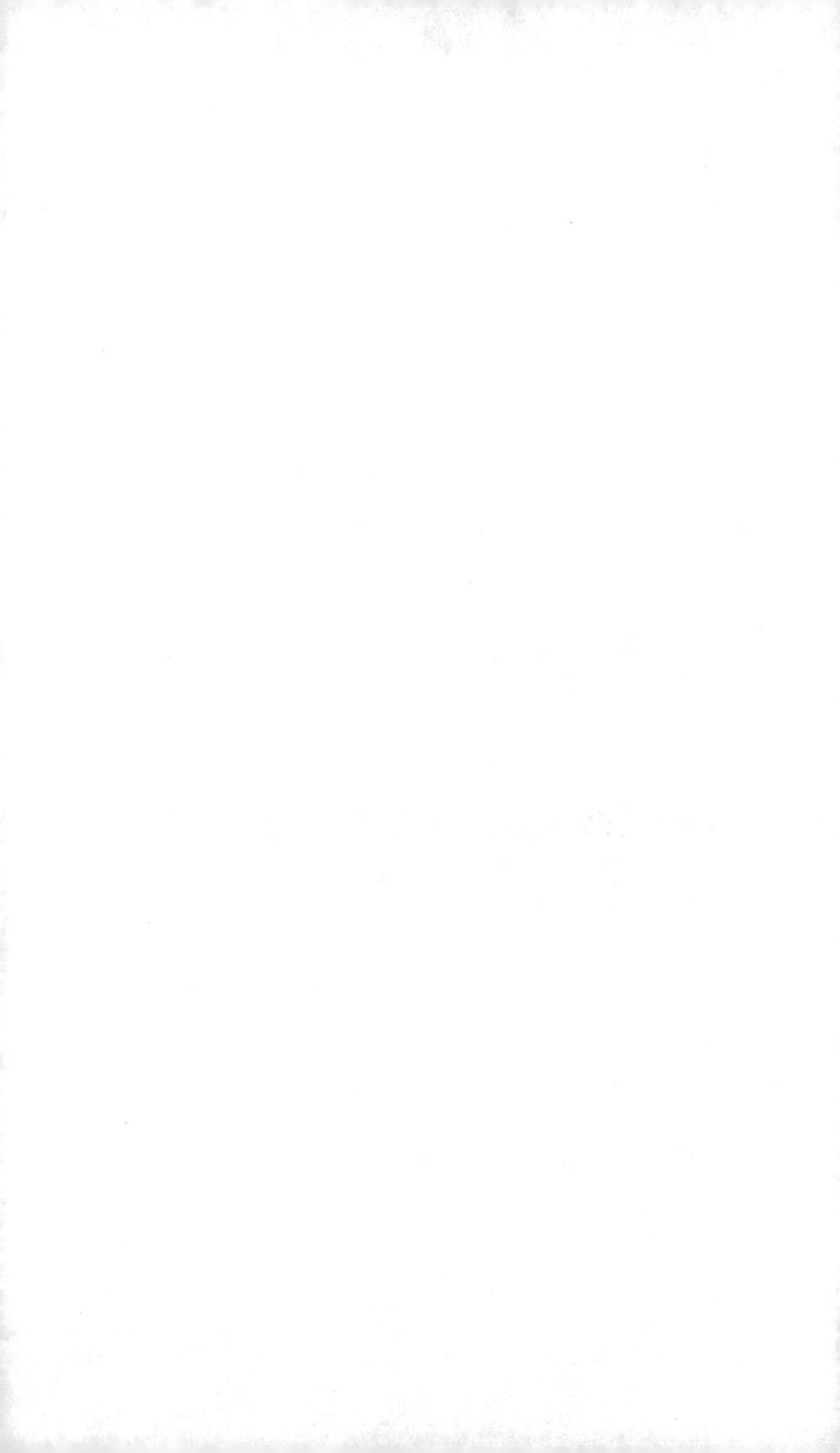

CHAPTER 7

FORGING THE CHAIN

Have no fear of perfection—you'll never reach it.
– Salvador Dalí

Hopefully by this point you have been trying to implement the changes from the previous chapters into your practice. If you have been working to bring your practice into alignment with your vision, it can be helpful to take a step back and assess your progress.

We've discussed the system as a chain of four links. Focused Leadership + Committed Team = Patient Loyalty + Greater Profitability. You have spent time forging those links into a strong chain that will dramatically improve all aspects of the practice. Remember that, unlike systems, this is a cultural change in the practice and, as long as you keep doing what you're doing, that culture will remain strong and sound. But what does it really *look* like? Is there an end point where you can say you've arrived? No, it's not a destination it's a journey and a never-ending journey at that. It's remarkable to me that the best practices I work with are those that stay with me for years and continue to beg the question of what more can be done. There's a saying that "the greatest enemy of being excellent is being good." For the top tier of dentists in the country, good is never enough.

Let's take a look at what the practice should *look* and *feel* like for the dentist, the team, and the patients when what we've discussed is being implemented.

I had a client who produced over $2 million annually tell me a story. We had been working on creating amazing patient experiences and one of the things we decided he should do was to call all his new patients the day before their appointment and say, "Hi, this is Dr. Mark, and I'm calling to welcome you to the practice and to find out if there is anything I need to know to make your visit more comfortable." What we found was that his new patients would not only show up for their appointments but they would keep future appointments, follow his treatment recommendations, and refer their friends and family. A colleague of his in the same small town asked him to what he attributed his success. My client told him how he made post-op calls and the colleague said, "Nah, I can't see myself doing that." Then he told him how he calls all his new patients and got the same response. The key was that my client was willing to do what most other practices aren't—and therein lies the difference. You can't be different unless you *do things differently.*

Worth Quoting

"If we can keep our competitors focused on us while we stay focused on the customer, ultimately we'll turn out all right."

Jeff Bezos

The Dentist

If anyone tries to tell you that this is easy for the doctor, they're greatly mistaken. Once you recognize and acknowledge this fact, things become easier because you realize that it's simply a question of applying basic fundamental principles every day. Improving your practice is hard work and you will need to be constantly vigilant, especially in the initial months, to ensure things do not slip back to the way they were because the downward pull of the status quo is lurking right over your shoulder behind you.

The late, great Jim Rohn had a wonderful story: What if you got the message of 'an apple a day' wrong? What if your story was a Snickers bar a day? If you jump on the scale tomorrow after eating a Snickers bar (250 calories) you probably won't notice any difference, however, if you jump back on the scale after a year of eating just one Snickers bar a day you will find that you will have eaten 91,250 extra calories and gained a whopping 26 pounds. That's the story behind Jim's famous quote which follows below. I have to say, this is my favorite quote of all time:

"Success is nothing more than a few simple disciplines practiced every day; while failure is a few errors in judgment repeated every day. It is the cumulative weight of either our disciplines or our judgments that leads to fortune or failure."

Here is what to do, step by step.

1. **Vision and Clarity of Direction:** Clarity is an empowering thing. The benefit of spending time defining your vision

statement is that you now have a clear picture of where you are going and how to get there. At this juncture, you should have a powerful vision statement and be working to align yourself and your team to do everything you can in support of it.

2. **Committed Team:** The ability to rely on your team makes all the difference and takes a huge weight off your shoulders. As we've discussed in the previous chapters, once a team is engaged and motivated, they'll be excited to help you achieve your goals, because your goals have become their goals as well. They'll be throwing their shoulder to the wheel right alongside you. Once everyone on the team has started to work toward the vision, the team will be collaborating and striving to set everyone else up for success.

3. **Less Management Time:** It became clear to me while doing the research for my first book (*What Do Dentists Really Want*), that managing staff is the one thing that stands clearly head and shoulders above all else when it comes to owning a dental practice. It can become such an immense source of stress that it can literally drive dentists to leave the profession. It isn't why you got into this business. As the dentist, you tend to have extreme focus on a very small area (a mouth is only about the size of an apple, after all!). There is no way you can know whether the receptionist is answering the phone like you want her to or whether the hygienist is really setting the stage with Mrs. Jones to do that crown. You should not have to worry about how the front desk person is interacting with patients or if the billing is being handled properly.

At this point, you as the dentist will be able to trust your team. You have set up the practice to run smoothly and there is no need for micro-managing them. Monitor, yes, but not micromanage.

4. **Predictability:** Holding your daily huddles and weekly staff meetings and monitoring the progress means that you will have predictable results. Your staff will be scheduling your appointments, handling last minute emergencies, and governing the flow of the day in such a way that you feel confident that your patients are being well taken care of and you don't feel stressed out.

5. **Fun at Work:** Seriously, you should be having fun. Now that the weight of tedious management tasks is off your shoulders, you should be able to relax and enjoy your job again. The relationship between yourself and the team, as well as between team members, should be relaxed and happy and everyone should be having fun and all the while working their hearts out. You'll find that patients begin to take note and start making comments about how much fun you seem to have in the practice and how much everyone likes each other. This makes for a more relaxed and fun visit for the patient and, believe me, it is not the norm in the dental industry.

6. **Increased Profitability:** Although this is the area many dentists initially care about, your hard work has not been directly related to profits. That being said, you should see an increase in profitability without even trying. Focusing simply on profit will, hopefully, get you just that, however, when you add focused leadership and a committed team into the mix, that's when profits

really begin to soar. One dentist I worked with told me that he was thrilled because he had been slaving away, six days a week, and barely getting by. Once he started implementing these principles, he saw a 25 percent increase in profitability, even though he himself was only working three and a half days a week. That's the kind of results you are looking for!

The Team

Every dental office is made up of team members, each serving a unique, but interconnected, function. There are receptionists, hygienists, financial coordinators, clinical assistants, and more— each must be performing their tasks to the best of their ability, but also focused on setting up the next person in the group for success. If you have managed to engage the team and align them with your vision, you should have a team that is collaborative, competent, and willing to go Above and Beyond. Here is what that looks like.

1. **Aligned With the Leader and Vision:** Your team is aligned with the vision you have established for the practice. If the vision has been properly reinforced with the team, each person will be mindful of consistently working towards achieving this vision. For them it becomes a 'bigger picture' scenario, one where it's not all about personal agendas or what's in it for me but rather about the *good of the practice*. In addition, the gap between the doctor and the staff is no longer getting in the way of team cohesiveness. There is no "us versus them" mentality—the whole office is a collective moving in the same direction. You'll find that by the time you've reached this stage

the team would never tolerate one of their own to be any less committed than they are. If a wrong hiring decision is made these people will quickly be weeded out.

2. **Shared Sense of Purpose:** This is hugely important and ties back to the first point. Many of the dental office employees I've worked with have arrived in the profession by chance. Dentistry was not their passion and chosen profession as it was for you. They may have just needed a job and answered an online ad. There's nothing wrong with that, but that can make it more difficult to feel engaged with your work. Teams that are motivated and aligned with the vision will have a shared sense of purpose. They have pride in what they do every day. This helps your team members feel that they have an important mission and an important part to play in their success and the success of the practice. The team knows that they are there to make a difference in people's lives. They can have a big impact on their patients, their co-workers and the practice as a whole and that makes them excited to come to work every morning.

3. **No Silos:** While it is important for employees to be skilled at their particular job function, an Above and Beyond Team must go beyond individual accomplishment. The members of the team should now be focused on how their actions impact other employees in the practice and since all the functions are interconnected, it is crucial that each member of the team consider how they can set the next team member up for success. So they do their jobs as well as they can, they appreciate the job being done by other members of the team and they will willingly step in to help where needed. Imagine a place where

there are no prima donna hygienists expecting a 'lowly' assistant to clean up after them. The culture dictates that, if there is a backlog in sterilization *everyone* steps in to help. Imagine if there is an unexpected opening in the schedule and the entire administrative team jumps in to help fill that opening. That's what it looks like to come out of your silo.

4. **Ability to Rely on One Another:** The result of team members setting each other up for success is that the staff will feel that they can rely on each other. No one wants to feel stressed out because they are not confident that the other parts of the process have not been performed properly. No one wants to pick up the pieces of someone else's mistakes. One of the biggest pet peeves for dentists is when they do not have the correct instruments on their tray when they sit down to begin a procedure. This slows down the treatment and makes them look disorganized in front of their patients. They get aggravated with the dental assistant, who in turn is embarrassed and flustered. In an Above and Beyond Team, this type of situation can be avoided and everyone can rely on one another. For instance, in the morning huddle, the team will discuss the patients coming in that day and the procedures that are going to be performed. They know if there are any special circumstances that need to be prepared for. The dentist can rely on his assistant to have everything ready when he sits down to work.

5. **Individual Strengths Development:** With a high functioning team you will find that everyone is looking for opportunities to grow both personally and professionally. You as the leader will naturally actively encourage and support their continuing education.

6. **Enjoyment and Fun:** Work should no longer be drudgery for the members of your team. People will not be just trying to make it through the day. If they are engaged and excited to make a difference at work, they will be challenging themselves to be the best they can be each day. Without the tensions and conflicts between the members of the team or the dentist, the Above and Beyond Team will actually enjoy being at work and have fun doing their jobs.

Worth Quoting

"If you work just for money, you'll never make it, but if you love what you're doing and you always put the customer first, success will be yours."

Ray Kroc, Founder, McDonalds

The Patients

We've already discussed how crucial improving patient loyalty is for your profitability. Loyalty comes from creating an amazing above and beyond experience with your office. The patients will notice the difference in your practice after you've worked to make the changes we've been talking about. Here's how your patients should feel.

1. **They Know My Name:** When a patient comes in, they are greeted personally by name. As part of the day's preparation, office staff will review patients and be sure they can identify

them. This seems trivial but it goes a long way towards making patients feel important to your office. Your patients will never have the experience of walking through the front door only to be met by people at the front desk clutching a phone to their ear and not even looking up. In your office, even though they may be in conversation they will look up and acknowledge you with a smile and indicate that they'll be with you shortly. Not only that but, even if you're a brand new patient, the assistant who comes to greet you in the reception room will walk right up to you and greet you by name.

2. **They're Warm and Friendly:** Your patients should always be treated with warmth and friendliness just like they were a family member. This helps your patients to feel at ease in a situation that could otherwise be one of high anxiety.

3. **They Know About Me Personally:** Your staff should remember personal details for each patient and include that in conversation with them. Imagine that you had a trip to Paris coming up last time you were in to visit your dentist. Now imagine the next time you come back they ask about your trip and perhaps ask to see some pictures. These things don't just happen because you have people with phenomenal memories but rather because you have put systems in place to make that sort of thing happen.

4. **They Treat Me Like Family But They Are Still Professional:** Patients should feel welcomed and valued when they come into the practice. But don't take that too far—you still want to come across as consummate professionals. Handle all business matters with professionalism and clarity so patients feel confident things are being handled properly.

5. **They Pay Attention to Detail:** The details matter. Make sure your staff pays attention to details so they come across to patients as being on top of everything. Notes should be made of any concerns patients express or any updates in terms of their contact or financial information. Be sure to always schedule follow up visits and contact them with timely reminders. Handle referrals to specialists, timely receipt of lab cases, and medical alerts and conditions with care. Your patients should feel confident all the details are being attended to without having to ask. One of the trademarks of your practice should be accuracy and attention to detail.

6. **There Are WOW Moments That Surprise and Delight Me:** In the chapter on patient loyalty, we discussed the WOW moments that you can incorporate into your practice. If you are doing several things in a consistent and meaningful way, your patients will notice. They will be delighted by these little gestures and will mention it to their friends. You want patients who say, "I have the best dentist! They do such fun, thoughtful things!"

Worth Quoting

"Aim for success, not perfection. Never give up your right to be wrong, because then you will lose the ability to learn new things and move forward with your life."

Dr. David M. Burns

Keep Working On It

Based on this assessment, take a close look at aspects that are not quite there yet. How can you keep making changes to help your practice go Above and Beyond? In the next chapter, we will examine more that can be done to keep your team motivated and on track.

Above and Beyond Action Items

Take a moment to evaluate how your practice looks and feels in the following areas.

Dentist
- Vision and Clarity of Direction
- Committed Team
- Less Management Time
- Predictability
- Fun at Work
- Increased Profitability

Team
- Aligned With The Leader and Vision
- Shared Sense of Purpose
- No Silos
- Ability to Rely on One Another
- Individual Strengths Development
- Enjoyment and Fun

Patients
- They Know My Name
- They Are Warm and Friendly
- They Know About Me Personally
- They Treat Me Like Family but Are Professional
- They Pay Attention to Detail
- There Are WOW Moments That Surprise and Delight Me

CHAPTER 8

KEEPING THE LINKS TOGETHER

Of course motivation is not permanent. But then, neither is bathing; that's why it is something you should do on a regular basis.

— Zig Ziglar

As you continue to make progress with creating an Above and Beyond Team, I want to stop to remind you of something. Changing course is *hard work,* but it's well worth the effort. It is a journey and you must accept that, at first, it will take a bit of hard work. The goal, however, is for the attitudes you are cultivating to become a way of life, to change the culture of your organization in a permanent, long-lasting way. With this cultural shift there is no doubt that your people will stay with you far longer than those in other practices and, when changes do take place or new people are added, they integrate into the culture around them. Once you have the momentum going and everyone operating at this new higher level, maintaining that momentum becomes much easier. It's sort of like a car: it takes much more gas to get to a certain speed than it does to maintain that speed.

Staying Motivated – The Team

You and your team need to find ways to remain motivated to maintain the high level of standards that you have achieved. Remember that problems in performance or attitude from members of your team ultimately rest with you. One practice I worked with discovered that their hygienists were over-reporting their reappointment rates on the tracking metric we set up. The dentists were appalled that their team members were being dishonest. I reminded them that this actually showed their team was not committed to the vision and that this was a problem of leadership that really came down to them as leaders. We worked on ways to motivate the staff so that they understood that their role in the team made it important to be accurate and honest; the hygienists desire to be a great part of the team led to actual high reappointment rates, thereby helping the entire practice.

Worth Quoting

"Motivation is what gets you started. Habit is what keeps you going."

Jim Rohn

Meetings: Use your meetings and huddles as a motivational tool by establishing them as "No Naysayer Zones." No one can say something "can't be done." Instead, everyone should be looking for creative and positive solutions to any issues that arise. Action item tasks should be assigned to achieve the next step in achieving the vision. Team members should be very clear on their individual responsibilities. At the end of each meeting, schedule the next one. That way, a deadline has been established for whatever has been assigned and everyone knows they are accountable for doing their tasks before the next meeting.

Share the Load: Make sure the responsibilities of the practice are being shared in a reasonable way so no one is overloaded. Just as the doctor cannot micromanage every aspect of the practice, neither can anyone else. Empower the members of your team to go Above and Beyond by setting each other up for success, to train those that need to be helped, and to do their jobs well because they care about the vision.

Recognizing and Rewarding The Team: When I say rewards, I don't necessarily mean financial ones. The biggest reward can be working in a place where they feel like they are doing a good job and making a difference. In an earlier chapter, I mentioned Ken Blanchard's book *Whale Done!* In this book he describes how trainers at Sea World have trained orca whales to perform using positive reinforcement. The same principles can be applied to workplace relationships to great effect. The key, Blanchard says, is to catch people doing things right and reward them for that. This need not be a huge accomplishment, but it should be specific and targeted. What do I mean by that? Don't thank everyone for a great day on the way out the door and think you've rewarded the team.

You must thank a specific person for a specific task. Here are some examples:

- If you have a well-balanced and seamless day, tell your receptionist/scheduler: "Thank you – you scheduled me the perfect day. Everything went so smoothly."
- If you have an assistant who is very helpful with a nervous patient, be sure to mention: "I noticed Mrs. Smith was terrified when she came back here and she walked out smiling. That was because of you. Thank you."
- The bottom line is important too, so if you notice your accounts receivable drops significantly, tell your accounts person: "I noticed you've been working hard to get our collections and accounts up to date. Thank you for that."

In addition to heartfelt thanks, random appreciation gifts to the whole team will surprise and delight them. Note that I said in addition – the specific praise is crucial to making your team feel motivated, but this type of reward will provide an added boost in morale. Perhaps treat everyone to coffee one morning or give everyone a goodie bag of spa products. Just a little something to brighten their day can make a big difference.

Staying Motivated – The Dentist

Here are some tips to help the dentist stay motivated throughout the process. We've touched on these things before, but maintaining enthusiasm and dedication to the vision is essential to your success.

Worth Quoting

"Most people give up just when they're about to achieve success. They quit on the one yard line. They give up at the last-minute of the game, one foot from a winning touchdown."

Ross Perot

Pace Yourself: If you ever attempted a massive project, you know it can be easy to become overwhelmed by the scope of it. Don't let the magnitude of the task get in your way. One of the keys to maintaining stamina and motivation for a large project is to pace yourself. Rome wasn't built in a day, and your Above and Beyond Team cannot be either.

Set manageable goals that break down the enormous tasks into smaller ones. This will allow you to take realistic steps that will move you closer to your overall goal. These small checklist victories will allow you to make progress without becoming burned out.

Here is a tool that works for me and it may be helpful for you as well. At the start of each day, I create a to-do list of action items. These can't be nebulous goals—each must be a clear thing that can be accomplished and checked off. I review the list and prioritize those that are most essential to do today. I highlight those and then number them in order of importance. That way, as I move through my day, once I check off one item, I know exactly what to tackle next.

I don't give myself the opportunity to ponder the list and, more than likely, get distracted by something else.

Lead By Example: We've discussed this before, but to motivate yourself and your team, you must commit publicly and visibly to the vision you have set forth. This is crucial to keeping your team motivated to stay the course with you. You must show you are leading by example and that you are on board with what you've told everyone else to do.

Why is this so important? I like the quote by Albert F. Schlieder: "We tend to judge others by their behavior and ourselves by our intentions." You may have this vision firmly in mind and so in your own estimation, you are doing well. But other people judge behavior—it doesn't matter what you are intending, it is what you actually do that counts. Make sure your intentions match your behavior so your team will know that it is important to you and therefore, should be important to them as well.

Reframe Your Thoughts: As you embark on this journey, you can expect resistance. People on the team will challenge you. This is unavoidable, but it is very important to avoid this negativity in your own thoughts. If someone on the team (or even your own mind) starts to say something along the lines of "this will never happen," reframe the discussion. Refer back to your to-do list. Talk about an actionable goal that *will* happen and celebrate a success that has been achieved. Negativity has no place in an Above and Beyond Team so do your best to change the conversation.

Stay the Course: While it is a useful tool to break up your tasks into manageable segments, you will do well to keep the end goal in mind.

The results you are striving for (an Above and Beyond Team, loyal patients, a profitable practice, an enjoyable workplace) will prove to be the most motivating thing to get you through the hard work.

Worth Quoting

"A man can be as great as he wants to be. If you believe in yourself and have the courage, the determination, the dedication, the competitive drive and if you are willing to sacrifice the little things in life and pay the price for the things that are worthwhile, it can be done."

Vince Lombardi

Above and Beyond

Remember that it starts with you making the decision that you will do whatever it takes to go Above and Beyond. More than anything, keeping the chain together comes down to your own resolve. You must decide where you want to go and the steps that will get there. But it is the "where" that will carry you through. If you have the end in mind, the other things you are hoping for will come to you as well.

If your goal is to have a great team that provides outstanding experiences, you will get loyal patients. Those loyal patients will lead to financial rewards. The financial rewards will allow you the freedom to enjoy your work again.

Remember my client from the first chapter? After we had been working together for a while, he took my hand and said to me, "All my success, I owe to you. I didn't like coming to work anymore. I didn't have time for my family. But now I am dialed in and I love coming to work every morning. Thank you so much."

You too can have that success! Are you ready to take your team Above and Beyond?

APPENDIX

Template for Promoting Change:

This is the blank template, please see below for a working example

Step 1: Establish the goal.	
Describe the situation as you would like to see it regardless of current conditions and constraints. Solicit and listen to ideas from the team. Write the goal down.	Date:

Step 2: Determine the Gaps.	
Establish the gap between where you are and where you need to go to reach the goal.	Date:

Step 3: Establish What Needs to be Done and By Whom.

List out every individual undertaking that needs to take place to reach the goal and determine who needs to do what.	Date:

Step 4: Monitor and Communicate Results.

Determine how results will be measured and communicated to the team.	Date:

List the team members who need to be involved:

Obtain verbal agreement from each of them:

Designate who is going to track and communicate the results (may be different people):

When and where will the results be communicated:

Step 5: Take Action and Make Minor Adjustments Along the Way.	
Begin the process of change with your committed team and be prepared to make some minor adjustments along the way.	Date:

How frequently will the team meet to discuss progress and determine if adjustments need to be made:

Which individuals have contributed the most?

How should incremental individual and collective successes be acknowledged?

Working Example of Template for Promoting Change:

Step 1: Establish the goal.	
Describe the situation as you would like to see it regardless of current conditions and constraints. Solicit and listen to ideas from the team. Write the goal down.	Date:
I'd like to see the administrators better able to identify patients when they walk through the door. I'd like to se the hygienists and assistants walk up to the patient in the reception room with confidence and invite them back into the treatment room.	

Step 2: Determine the Gaps.	
Establish the gap between where you are and where you need to go to reach the goal.	Date:
Currently the administrators don't proactively attempt to recognize who is walking through the front door by immediately looking up, smiling and, whenever possible, greeting them by name. The assistants and hygienists stand in the doorway to the reception room and call the patients' name. I want the to be able to go directly to the patient, with confidence, and greet them and invite them to come back with them.	

Step 3: Establish What Needs to be Done and By Whom.

List out every individual undertaking that needs to take place to reach the goal and determine who needs to do what.	Date:

ADMIN:
1. Get a camera that can be linked to the computer and take pictures of all patients
2. Review the patients ahead of time so that you can remember their faces
3. As soon as they walk through the door, look up, smile and say something like: "Hi Mr. Smith. It's so good to see you again! Please have a seat and I'll let them know you're here. They shouldn't be more than 5 minutes. Can I get you a cup of coffee?"
4. If it is likely that a new patient is the one you're expecting, say something like "You must be Mr. Smith, I'm so glad to meet you. My name is Sally, we spoke on the phone yesterday. Welcome to the practice."
5. Send a note to the assistants or hygienists describing what Mr. Smith is wearing or some other distinguishing feature or even where he is sitting.

ASSISTANTS/HYGIENISTS:
1. Before going out to collect your patient, check the picture in the computer and check to see what the patient's descriptor or distinguishing feature is or where they're sitting.
2. Walk confidently right up to the patient in the reception. Smile, maintain great eye contact and invite them to follow you.
3. Verbiage for existing patient: "Mr. Smith, it's great seeing you again. Please, come on back, we're ready for you."
4. Verbiage for new patient: "Mr. Smith, it is so nice to meet you, my name is Sally and I'm Doctor's assistant/hygienist. Please come on back, we're ready for you.

Step 4: Monitor and Communicate Results.	
Determine how results will be measured and communicated to the team.	Date:

List the team members who need to be involved:
Suzie: Receptionist
Rachel: Hygienist
Mary: Hygienist
Julie: Assistant
Amber: Assistant

Obtain verbal agreement from each of them:
Suzie: Done 4/1/13
Rachel: Done 4/1/13
Mary: Done 4/1/13
Julie: Done 4/1/13
Amber: Done 4/1/13

Designate who is going to track and communicate the results (may be different people):
Suzie will keep track and give feedback
Sandy (OM) will keep track for Suzie and give feedback
Suzie will keep track and give feedback for the assistants and hygienists

When and where will the results be communicated:
Discuss how things are going, give feedback, suggestions and, above all, praise during huddles and staff meetings

Step 5: Take Action and Make Minor Adjustments Along the Way.	
Begin the process of change with your committed team and be prepared to make some minor adjustments along the way.	Date:

How frequently will the team meet to discuss progress and determine if adjustments need to be made:
Informal discussions daily in the huddle
Add as an agenda item to staff meetings

Which individuals have contributed the most?
TBD

How should incremental individual and collective successes be acknowledged?
Individual praise from myself, Suzie and Sandy. Above all, look for improvement, not perfection initially. Acknowledge by describing specifically what was seen and, when needed, give feedback and encouragement.

When everybody feels like they're batting 100, let's schedule lunch out as a group to celebrate

Patient Satisfaction Survey

Your opinion really matters and your input, both positive and negative, is always taken into account. Please complete the survey regarding our practice.

Please let us know how we did.	Poor	Fair	Good	Very Good	Excellent
How long did you have to wait to make an appointment?	p	p	p	p	p
How long did you have to wait in the reception area?	p	p	p	p	p
Explanation of treatment received?	p	p	p	p	p
Explanation of treatment recommended?	p	p	p	p	p
Technical skills of the health-care provider you saw? (Clinical skills, thoroughness, carefulness, competence)	p	p	p	p	p
Explanation of financial options?	p	p	p	p	p
Personal manner of clinical team? (Friendliness, customer service, respect, sensitivity)	p	p	p	p	p
Personal manner of front office team? (Friendliness, customer service, respect, sensitivity)	p	p	p	p	p
The overall visit?	p	p	p	p	p

What and/or who stood out to you either positive or negative?
Do you have any additional feedback or ideas on what we can do to deliver an Above and Beyond patient experience?

Patient Survey

Dear Patient,

Here at _____, we do not want to be ordinary. We don't want to give you what you could get anywhere else. We want to provide the patients who choose our office with not only exceptional dentistry but also extraordinary service.

It is probably apparent to you that some serious thought goes into choosing the people that I entrust to serve you. From time to time, it's important to check in with you, the patient, to find out what we're doing right and, most importantly, what we could be doing better. Please take a moment of your time to let us know how we're doing. Please know that my door is always open if you ever need to speak to me personally. If it is a private matter, please feel free to call me at my home at _____

Sincerely,

1. Did we answer the phone pleasantly?   ❏ Yes ❏ No

2. Were you greeted by our receptionist within
a few moments of entering?   ❏ Yes ❏ No

3. Was your wait in the reception room
reasonably short?   ❏ Yes ❏ No

4. Was the reception room clean and comfortable?   ❏ Yes ❏ No

5. Was your treatment in our office comfortable?   ❏ Yes ❏ No

6. Did we explain your needed dental
treatment and fees to your satisfaction?   ❏ Yes ❏ No

7. Was the clinical team pleasant and
helpful to you during treatment?   ❏ Yes ❏ No

8. What did you like best about our office? _____

_____

9. Was there anything you did not like about our office? _____

_____

10. Was there any team member who
    stood out to you?   ❏ Good ❏ Bad

If so, why?_____

_____ Signed (Optional)

Welcome Letter for Adult New Patients

Date

Name

Address

Dear Patient,

Welcome to our office! We appreciate the confidence and trust you have placed in us and look forward to meeting you personally.

Our philosophy of care governs everything we do for our patients:

☆ We truly care about our patients and strive to provide an exceptional experience for each and every patient in our office.

☆ We treat every patient as an individual and our goal is to help you to retain your teeth in comfort, function and aesthetics for the rest of your life.

☆ We work hard to explain treatment in detail to you and to provide the most accurate fee estimate possible.

☆ Whenever possible we will phase treatment for you according to your time and financial constraints.

At your first visit, we will take the time to get to know you (and you, us) and discuss your dental needs and desires. We will perform a comprehensive dental evaluation and gather information to make a customized treatment plan for you.

Enclosed you will find our new patient information forms. Please fill these out and bring them with you to your first appointment along with your insurance card (if applicable) and a list of any medications you take.

We are looking forward to meeting you!

Sincerely,

Team Satisfaction Survey

Your opinion really matters and your input, both positive and negative, is always taken into account. Please complete the survey regarding our practice.

	Strongly Disagree	Some-what Disagree	Neutral	Some-what Agree	Strongly Agree
I have the opportunity to participate in the goal setting process?	p	p	p	p	p
I am given adequate feedback regarding my performance.	p	p	p	p	p
I get praise and recognition when I do a good job.	p	p	p	p	p
Teamwork is encouraged and practiced in this organization.	p	p	p	p	p
This practice is extremely focused on patients' needs.	p	p	p	p	p
We constantly look for ways in which to improve.	p	p	p	p	p
I have a good understanding of the mission and goals of the practice.	p	p	p	p	p
I understand how my work directly contributes to the overall success of the practice.	p	p	p	p	p
My salary is competitive with similar jobs I might find elsewhere.	p	p	p	p	p

	Strongly Disagree	Some-what Disagree	Neutral	Some-what Agree	Strongly Agree
My work is challenging, stimulating and rewarding.	⊓	⊓	⊓	⊓	⊓
The amount of work I am asked to do is reasonable.	⊓	⊓	⊓	⊓	⊓
I am treated fairly in this practice.	⊓	⊓	⊓	⊓	⊓
Our leader/s lead by example.	⊓	⊓	⊓	⊓	⊓
My leader values my talents and the contribution I make.	⊓	⊓	⊓	⊓	⊓
My coworkers care about me as a person.	⊓	⊓	⊓	⊓	⊓
This practice has high performance standards.	⊓	⊓	⊓	⊓	⊓
People are held accountable for achieving goals and meeting expectations.	⊓	⊓	⊓	⊓	⊓
My workplace is a physically comfortable place to work.	⊓	⊓	⊓	⊓	⊓
Communication is encouraged in this practice.	⊓	⊓	⊓	⊓	⊓
I am comfortable sharing my opinions at work.	⊓	⊓	⊓	⊓	⊓
Senior management is genuinely interested in employee opinions and ideas.	⊓	⊓	⊓	⊓	⊓
I love my job.	⊓	⊓	⊓	⊓	⊓

Additional comments, thoughts and ideas:

Practice Health Assessment Tool

Your opinion really matters and your input, both positive and negative, is always taken into account. Please complete the survey regarding our practice.

Practice Health Assessment Tool	Strongly Disagree	Some-what Disagree	Neutral	Some-what Agree	Strongly Agree
We always greet our patients by name.	☐	☐	☐	☐	☐
We rarely keep our patients waiting.	☐	☐	☐	☐	☐
Our patients always know their fees for upcoming treatment.	☐	☐	☐	☐	☐
We explain treatment thoroughly.	☐	☐	☐	☐	☐
We constantly look for ways in which to improve.	☐	☐	☐	☐	☐
We give our patients treatment options whenever possible.	☐	☐	☐	☐	☐
Our treatment plans are accurate and clear.	☐	☐	☐	☐	☐
We almost never make mistakes and, when we do, we immediately apologize.	☐	☐	☐	☐	☐
We always make postop calls to our patients.	☐	☐	☐	☐	☐
We work well together as a team.	☐	☐	☐	☐	☐
We have a good leader.	☐	☐	☐	☐	☐

Practice Health Assessment Tool	Strongly Disagree	Some-what Disagree	Neutral	Some-what Agree	Strongly Agree
We seldom experience conflict and gossiping.	☐	☐	☐	☐	☐
Our team is friendly and professional.	☐	☐	☐	☐	☐
Our doctor/s have a great bedside manner with patients.	☐	☐	☐	☐	☐
Our facility and surroundings are clean and appealing.	☐	☐	☐	☐	☐
Our patients are fiercely loyal.	☐	☐	☐	☐	☐
Our patients are happy to refer their family, friends and co-workers.	☐	☐	☐	☐	☐
We perform at a high level.	☐	☐	☐	☐	☐

Additional comments, thoughts and ideas:

ABOUT THE AUTHOR

Janet Steward is president of Janet Steward Consulting, a national firm focused on growing practices through team motivation that drives patient loyalty, which ultimately results in greater profitability.

She holds memberships to the Academy for Professional Speaking, Academy of Dental Management Consultants, the Speaking Consultant Network, the Institute of Management Consultants, Toastmasters International, and she is also a Certified Professional Behavior Analyst.

After studying business at the University of Cape Town in South Africa and immigrating to the United States in 1986, Janet began her career in dental practice management. She started her own consulting business, Janet Steward Consulting, in 2003 and has helped hundreds of dentists make their dreams for their practices become a reality. Janet speaks nationally and she is a high energy and engaging. She has a fun, approachable style and charms her audiences with her accent and her entertaining stories to help illustrate key points in her presentations.

She has been published nationwide, and she authored another book titled *What Do Dentists Really Want? Macromanage Your Way to Greater Freedom and a Million-Dollar Practice.* She can be contacted at Janet@janetstewardconsulting.com or 970-207-0776.